Better Homes and Gardens®

3 STEPS TO WEIGHT LOSS

Better Homes and Gardens® Books
Des Moines, Iowa

S

Better Homes and Gardens® Books
An imprint of Meredith® Books

3 Steps to Weight Loss
Editor: Jan Miller, R.D.
Associate Art Director: Mick Schnepf
Contributing Editors: Spectrum Communication Services, Inc., Marcia Stanley, M.S., R.D., Mary Williams
Contributing Writers: Lawrence J. Cheskin, M.D., Laurie Friedman Donze, Ph.D., Deborah Ezell, M.S., Lorraine Giangrandi, R.D., L.D.
Copy Chief: Terri Fredrickson
Managers, Book Production: Pam Kvitne, Marjorie J. Schenkelberg
Contributing Copy Editor: Daniel Cubias
Contributing Proofreaders: Maria Duryee, Jacquelyn Foster, Gretchen Kauffman, Carolyn Petersen
Photographers: Robert Jacobs, Scott Little
Food Stylists: Dianna Nolin, Charles Worthington
Indexer: Kathleen Poole
Electronic Production Coordinator: Paula Forest
Editorial and Design Assistants: Judy Bailey, Mary Lee Gavin, Karen Schirm
Test Kitchen Director: Lynn Blanchard
Test Kitchen Product Supervisor: Marilyn Cornelius

Meredith® Books
Editor in Chief: James D. Blume
Design Director: Matt Strelecki
Managing Editor: Gregory H. Kayko
Executive Food Editor: Jennifer Dorland Darling

Director, Retail Sales and Marketing: Terry Unsworth
Director, Sales, Special Markets: Rita McMullen
Director, Sales, Premiums: Michael A. Peterson
Director, Sales, Retail: Tom Wierzbicki
Director, Book Marketing: Brad Elmitt
Director, Operations: George A. Susral
Director, Production: Douglas M. Johnston

Vice President, General Manager: Jamie L. Martin

Better Homes and Gardens® Magazine
Editor in Chief: Jean LemMon
Executive Food Editor: Nancy Byal

Meredith Publishing Group
President, Publishing Group: Stephen M. Lacy
Vice President, Finance and Administration: Max Runciman

Meredith Corporation
Chairman and Chief Executive Officer: William T. Kerr

Chairman of the Executive Committee: E. T. Meredith III

Our seal assures you that every recipe in *3 Steps to Weight Loss* has been tested in the Better Homes and Gardens® Test Kitchen. This means that each recipe is practical and reliable, and meets our high standards of taste appeal. We guarantee your satisfaction with this book for as long as you own it.

All of us at Better Homes and Gardens® Books are dedicated to providing you with the information and ideas you need to create delicious foods. We welcome your comments and suggestions. Write to us at: Better Homes and Gardens Books, Cookbook Editorial Department, 1716 Locust St., Des Moines, IA 50309-3023.

If you would like to purchase any of our cooking, crafts, gardening, home improvement, or home decorating and design books, check wherever quality books are sold. Or visit us at: bhgbooks.com.

Pictured on front cover: Roast Tarragon Chicken (see recipe, page 94) Photographer: Robert Jacobs, Food Stylist: Charles Worthington

Contents.

foreword.

Based on my experience at Johns Hopkins Weight Management Center, the key to long-term, permanent weight loss is a complete program that includes all of the areas that influence weight—diet, behavior, and exercise. With the input of experts who work with me at Johns Hopkins, we've created a unique plan based on a nutritious but satisfying diet. This is not a traditional diet book containing hundreds of pages of text and advice; the basic plan is described in the first 12 pages of the book. Neither is it a traditional cookbook. Instead you will find a weight loss plan tailored for your specific body size. The book features tips for making positive lifestyle changes, guidelines for becoming more active, and more than 100 recipes to enjoy while losing those unwanted pounds.

My thanks go to the entire staff at the Johns Hopkins Weight Management Center and especially to the experts who helped me to write this book: Laurie Friedman Donze, Ph.D., for the behavioral information, Deborah Ezell, M.S., for the exercise guide; and Lorraine Giangrandi, R.D., L.D., C.N.S.D., for her nutritional knowledge. I would also like to acknowledge the invaluable help of Jan Miller, R.D. at Meredith® Books for her input and guidance, and the home economists in the Better Homes and Gardens® Test Kitchen responsible for countless hours of experimentation with recipes designed to make healthful dining both a pleasurable and satisfying experience.

Lawrence J. Cheskin, M.D.

Lawrence Cheskin, MD

Director of the Weight Management
Center at Johns Hopkins University

GETTING READY:

In the following pages you will find three simple steps to weight loss: 1. Find your desirable weight, 2. Determine how many calories you need to eat to lose, and 3. Follow a healthy eating plan designed to help take off the pounds. Because successful weight loss plans usually require lifestyle changes, you will also find helpful hints for making these changes easier, ways to reward your progress, and tips for becoming more active. Before you begin this healthy eating plan and embark on the journey to a new, thinner you, let's do a little soul-searching.

How Ready Are You?

So you want to lose weight. Are you really ready? Based on our experience at the Johns Hopkins Weight Management Center, individuals who are not ready to lose weight have a difficult time making the lifestyle changes that are important for weight loss.

What are your main reasons for wanting to lose weight?

_____ To improve my appearance

_____ To improve my health or reduce my risk of medical problems

_____ To improve my energy level or fitness

_____ To please someone important to me

_____ To look good for an upcoming event

_____ To improve some other area of my life (e.g.: find a partner, get a better job)

Obviously, if you can't identify any reasons to lose weight, doing so will be difficult! However, if you checked one or more, think about your reasons and consider these questions:

ONE Are your reasons specific? A vague reason such as "It's a good idea" is likely to be less motivating than one that applies specifically to you.

TWO Are they important to you? Your reasons might be great ones, but if they don't really matter to you, they won't be motivating.

THREE Do they require immediate results? Improving your health is a likely outcome of weight loss, but you may not see these results right away.

FOUR Do they meet your needs and not just the needs of others? Losing weight must be important to _you_. If you're taking on this mission primarily to please someone else, it won't keep you motivated enough to meet your goals. As selfish as it sounds, do this just for you!

FIVE Can they sustain your motivation over the long term? Losing weight for an upcoming wedding or other special occasion may motivate you until the big event, but what happens afterward? Similarly, many people expect certain changes following weight loss, such as a busier social life or new job opportunities. If these expected life improvements don't follow weight loss, motivation tends to dwindle.

Which Factors May Interfere with Your Ability to Stick to a Weight Loss Plan?

____Lack of time. As with most worthwhile things, following a healthy eating plan may take time and effort. Learning the ins and outs of a meal plan will initially require a little time. You will need time to prepare meals so that you aren't vulnerable to the convenience of fast food, and time for regular physical activity.

____Lack of support from your partner, family, or others. Friends and family members may not support you simply because they don't know _how_ to support you. On the other hand, if a family member or other individual seems to be deliberately sabotaging your efforts, you need to be assertive and set limits with this person. If the saboteur is your spouse or partner, you should discuss whether he/she feels threatened by your weight loss.

____Major stressful event(s). Major life changes or stress in your life—work (job changes), finances, relationships (marriage, divorce), residence (moving), school (beginning or ending), children (birth or parenting issues), death or loss, or a serious illness—could make weight loss difficult.

____Presence of an untreated psychological or psychiatric problem. Depression, anxiety, an eating disorder, or similar problems can be debilitating and painful, and they will surely interfere with your weight loss attempt. If you think you have psychological issues, seek advice from a qualified professional.

Even with a great plan and the best intentions, if you are experiencing any of these stresses, they may be roadblocks to your success. Evaluate your current lifestyle and make any necessary changes to ensure that you are ready to stick your plan.

Three Steps

One. Check Your Weight

Remember looking up your weight on the old height and weight tables to see if you were overweight? Well, those old tables based on life insurance company statistics have fallen out of favor because they do not reflect the actual risk for the average American. Instead, a measure called body-mass index (BMI) is now widely accepted as the standard measure of weight adjusted for height. Rather than evaluating absolute body weight, BMI is a ratio of your weight to height. People with a higher BMI tend to have a higher risk of developing long-term health problems. Although, if you are muscular, you may have a high BMI without any additional health risks.

To determine your BMI, consult the table on page 8. A BMI of 19 to 24.9 is considered healthy, 25 to 30 is considered overweight, and 30 or higher is considered obese. Find your height in the left-hand column and move across to find your weight; look to see what category you fall into.

The decision to attempt to lose weight if you fall into the overweight or obese category by BMI is up to you, as the table is only a guideline. In fact, one of the limitations of the current knowledge of obesity is that it is difficult to accurately predict who will suffer a health complication from being overweight and who won't. Family and personal histories provide some guidance. If overweight close relatives have suffered from heart disease at a relatively early age, or have type 2 (adult-onset) diabetes, it could mean a higher risk for you. If you personally have one of the health conditions commonly associated with obesity, including high cholesterol, high blood pressure, diabetes, or heart

Step One. Check Your Weight

WEIGHT (POUNDS)													
	HEALTHY BMI: 19-24.9						OVERWEIGHT BMI: 25-30					OBESE BMI: >30	
4′10″	91	96	100	105	110	115	119	124	129	134	138	143	167	191
4′11″	94	99	104	109	114	119	124	128	133	138	143	148	173	198
5′0″	97	102	107	112	118	123	128	133	138	143	148	153	179	204
5′1″	100	106	111	116	122	127	132	137	143	148	153	158	185	211
5′2″	104	109	115	120	126	131	136	142	147	153	158	164	191	218
5′3″	107	113	118	124	130	135	141	146	152	158	163	169	197	225
5′4″	110	116	122	128	134	140	145	151	157	163	169	174	204	232
5′5″	114	120	126	132	138	144	150	156	162	168	174	180	210	240
5′6″	118	124	130	136	142	148	155	161	167	173	179	186	216	247
5′7″	121	127	134	140	146	153	159	166	172	178	185	191	223	255
5′8″	125	131	138	144	151	158	164	171	177	184	190	197	230	262
5′9″	128	135	142	149	155	162	169	176	182	189	196	203	236	270
5′10″	132	139	146	153	160	167	174	181	188	195	202	207	243	278
5′11″	136	143	150	157	165	172	179	186	193	200	208	215	250	286
6′0″	140	147	154	162	169	177	184	191	199	206	213	221	258	294
6′1″	144	151	159	166	174	182	189	197	201	212	219	227	265	302
6′2″	148	155	163	171	179	186	194	202	210	218	225	233	272	311
6′3″	152	160	168	176	184	192	200	208	216	224	232	240	279	319
6′4″	156	164	172	180	189	197	205	213	221	230	238	246	287	328

disease, your risk of further problems such as a heart attack or stroke is increased, particularly if you are overweight or obese.

What's Your Goal?

Your goal weight should be realistic and achievable for who you are today (not 25 years ago!).

For example, if you haven't weighed less than 155 pounds since you were 16, a goal weight of 120 pounds may be unrealistic. Instead of setting a goal that you can't reach, choose a more reasonable goal, such as the lowest adult weight that you have maintained for a year or more. If this goal weight doesn't seem satisfying, it might still be a good initial goal. Once you reach this first goal, take a step back and reevaluate how you feel. Decide whether you want to set a lower goal weight and continue with weight loss. Keep in mind that most of the health benefits of weight loss can be achieved with a small amount of weight loss (5 to 10 percent of your initial body weight). You don't have to have a healthy BMI to experience a positive effect on your health. For example, a 200-pound, 5-foot-6-inch woman would still be considered overweight at 180 pounds (a 10 percent weight loss), but she would have a substantially lower risk for health problems.

As you track your weight loss, resist the temptation to jump on the scale more than once a day. Weigh yourself daily, at the same time, wearing the same amount of clothing. Take day-to-day fluctuations in stride, but if the scale shows an upward trend over a few weeks, it's best addressed.

Two. What You Need to Live

Everyone is unique. Height, weight, and daily physical activity vary from person to person. Even if you are the same height and weight as a friend, your calorie needs may be higher or lower due to differing activity levels. For best results, you need to know how many calories you need to lose weight. Match your weight in the left column of the table on page 10 with the activity level that best describes your lifestyle. Write down the corresponding number of calories.

Refer to your results from Step One and get ready to do a little math. If you are at a healthy weight, this is the amount of calories you need to maintain your weight. If you are overweight, subtract 500 calories from your daily needs. If you are obese, subtract 750 calories from your daily needs.

For example, if you are a 5-foot 7-inch woman who weighs 180 pounds (a BMI considered to be overweight) and have the activity level of a Couch Spud, you need 2,340 calories per day to maintain your weight. Because you fall into the overweight category, subtract 500 calories to give you a total of 1,840 calories to promote weight loss.

If you are a 6-foot 3-inch male who weighs 190 pounds (a BMI in the healthy category) and have a Fairly Brisk activity level, you need 3,135 calories to maintain your healthy weight.

To determine activity levels choose the category that best describes you:

Couch Spud: *Mainly sitting all day, standing, reading, or typing* **Go-Lightly:** *Walking is the main exercise, but no more than 2 hours a day* **Fairly Brisk:** *Heavy housework, gardening, and brisk walking (about a 15-minute mile)* **Very Active:** *Labor-intensive job or vigorous daily exercise such as running*

Step Two. What You Need to Live

Women's Daily Calorie Needs

Weight	Couch Spud	Go-Lightly	Fairly Brisk	Very Active
100	1,300	1,400	1,500	1,600
110	1,430	1,540	1,650	1,760
120	1,560	1,680	1,800	1,920
130	1,690	1,820	1,950	2,080
140	1,680	1,960	2,100	2,240
150	1,950	2,100	2,250	2,400
160	2,080	2,240	2,400	2,560
170	2,210	2,380	2,550	2,720
180	2,340	2,520	2,700	2,880
190	2,470	2,660	2,850	3,040
200	2,600	2,800	3,000	3,200
210	2,730	2,940	3,150	3,360
220	2,860	3,080	3,300	3,520

Men's Daily Calorie Needs

Weight	Couch Spud	Go-Lightly	Fairly Brisk	Very Active
150	2,145	2,310	2,475	2,640
160	2,288	2,464	2,640	2,816
170	2,431	2,618	2,805	2,992
180	2,574	2,772	2,970	3,168
190	2,717	2,926	3,135	3,344
200	2,860	3,080	3,300	3,520
210	3,003	3,234	3,465	3,696
220	3,146	3,388	3,630	3,872
230	3,289	3,542	3,795	4,048
240	3,432	3,696	3,960	4,224
250	3,575	3,850	4,125	4,400
260	3,718	4,004	4,290	4,576

Three. Your Daily Eating Plan

After you've determined your calorie goal based on the tables from page 10, find the correct Daily Eating Plan on page 12 to help you lose weight or maintain a healthy diet. Use the Food List on page 13 as a guide for portion sizes in each group.

Flex Your Plan

Your meal plan can be as flexible as your lifestyle demands. Divide the total number of food group servings by the number of meals and snacks you typically eat in a day. If you usually eat one to two meals per day, consider the following tips for a more healthful approach:

Don't skip meals. It is best to eat three meals and one to two snacks each day. Eating small amounts throughout the day helps reduce hunger, especially when cutting back on calories. You'll be less tempted to overeat to make up for that skipped meal. This doesn't mean you should always eat three full meals every day whether you are hungry or not. A light meal or snack might satisfy you when you aren't very hungry.

Watch the soda! It is easy to unknowingly drink extra calories if you sip high-calorie beverages such as soda or fruit juice throughout the day. Even though you eat a fairly healthful diet with reasonable portion sizes, the calories from regular soda and high-calorie juice drinks can put you over the top and contribute to weight gain. Soda doesn't give your body any nutrients, only calories. Fruit juice, although it is more nutrient-dense, can pack a lot of calories in a small amount. A serving of juice is rather small—$3/_4$ cup. When you include juice in your meal plan, don't drink more than one to two servings each day. A piece of raw fruit is a better choice because it is usually portioned and provides your body with fiber that helps to keep you full. Whole milk, another nutrient-dense beverage, is also high in calories and fat. Gradually switching to fat-free milk reduces the calories and fat in your diet without decreasing the calcium.

Dining Out

Your meal plan can easily accommodate a dinner out if you plan wisely. If dining out is part of your daily routine, keep these tips in mind:

1. Plan a light dinner if you ate a big lunch.
2. Decide ahead of time to skip dessert.
3. Order an appetizer and make it a meal.
4. Select the types and amounts of food that best fit your plan and stick to them without succumbing to temptations. Restaurant portions are often generous. Follow the portion sizes recommended in the Food Lists on page 13 or split your dinner with a friend.
5. Being a member of "The Clean Plate Club" is not mandatory.
6. Ask how the food is prepared. Choose foods that are cooked with the "B" methods, that is baked, broiled, boiled, or braised.
7. Order sauces and salad dressings on the side so you can better control your calorie intake.

1,200-1,500 Calories

Food Group	Number of servings	Calories per serving	Fat per serving (grams)
Bread/Cereal/Rice/Pasta	5	80	0-3
Vegetables	4	25	0
Fruits	2	60	0
Milk/Milk Products	3	100	0-5
Meat/Meat Substitutes	2	110	0-6
Fats, Oils, and Sweets	2	50	0-5

1,500-1,800 Calories

Bread/Cereal/Rice/Pasta	6	80	0-3
Vegetables	4	25	0
Fruits	3	60	0
Milk/Milk Products	3	100	0-5
Meat/Meat Substitutes	3	110	0-6
Fats, Oils, and Sweets	3	50	0-5

1,800-2,100 Calories

Bread/Cereal/Rice/Pasta	9	80	0-3
Vegetables	4	25	0
Fruits	3	60	0
Milk/Milk Products	3	100	0-5
Meat/Meat Substitutes	3	110	0-6
Fats, Oils, and Sweets	4	50	0-5

2,100-2,400 Calories

Bread/Cereal/Rice/Pasta	10	80	0-3
Vegetables	5	25	0
Fruits	4	60	0
Milk/Milk Products	3	100	0-5
Meat/Meat Substitutes	4	110	0-6
Fats, Oils, and Sweets	4	50	0-5

A minimum of 12 grams of fat is a daily requirement for health and absorption of vitamins A, D, E, and K.

Food List*

Starch: Bread/Cereal/Rice/Pasta and Starchy Vegetables

½ cup dry cereal (high-fiber)
½ whole wheat pita
½ English muffin
½ cup cooked beans, peas, or lentils
½ cup cooked cereal, pasta, or rice
⅓ cup cooked couscous
¾ oz. pretzels
1 slice whole grain bread
2 slices reduced-calorie bread
6-inch flour or corn tortilla
3 graham crackers
5 whole wheat crackers
15-20 fat-free snack chips
½ cup sweet potato
⅓ cup baked beans
½ cup corn
1 small or ½ large baked potato

Vegetables

1 cup torn leafy greens:
    lettuce, spinach, romaine
1 cup raw vegetables:
    carrots, celery, bean sprouts,
    pea pods, tomato, or cucumber
½ cup cooked vegetables:
    broccoli, carrots, asparagus, green
    beans, zucchini, peppers, artichoke
    hearts, Brussels sprouts, eggplant

Fruit

6 oz. 100% fruit juice
1 mango or papaya
1 cup strawberries or raspberries
¾ cup blueberries or fresh pineapple
½ cup fresh cherries
1 medium banana
1 medium apple or pear
1 medium orange or grapefruit
¼ of a medium cantaloupe
½ cup honeydew melon
1¼ cups watermelon
1 kiwifruit, peach, or nectarine
2 small plums

Meat/Meat Substitute

2 oz. turkey or chicken (skinless, white
    meat), lean red meat (at least 90% lean),
    lean pork (Canadian bacon, tenderloin,
    fresh ham), or roasted lamb
2 oz. duck or pheasant (without skin)
3 oz. crab, tuna, or broiled fish
½ cup cottage cheese
2 eggs or ½ to ¾ cup egg substitute
4 oz. (½ cup) tofu

Milk/Milk Products

1 cup fat-free, reduced-fat milk or soy
    milk
1½ to 2 oz. fat-free or reduced-fat cheese
1 cup unsweetened or artificially sweetened
    yogurt

Fat, Oils, and Sweets

3 Tbsp. reduced-fat sour cream
2 Tbsp. jelly or preserves
2 Tbsp. reduced-calorie salad dressing
2 Tbsp. reduced-fat cream cheese
1 Tbsp. margarine or reduced-fat butter
1 Tbsp. regular dressing
1 Tbsp. sesame seeds
1 Tbsp. reduced-fat mayonnaise
2 tsp. peanut butter
1 tsp. oil (canola, olive, or peanut)
8 black olives
6 almonds or cashews
10 peanuts

Free Foods

Bouillon
Mustard
Salsa
Soy Sauce
Lemon or Lime Juice
Coffee and Tea
Diet Soft Drinks
Club Soda
Sugar-Free Tonic Water
Sugar-Free Gum

What's a Portion?

Typical size　　**Ideal size**

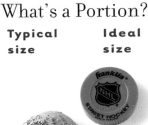
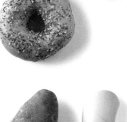
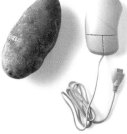

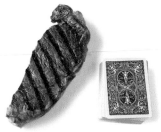
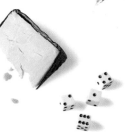

Portions are based on Food Guide Pyramid serving recommendations

Food Guide Pyramid

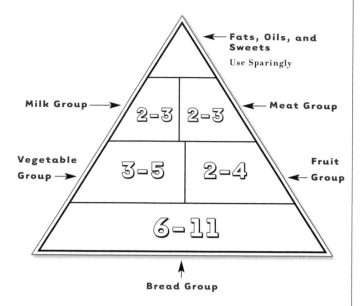

Good Nutrition

What is a good diet anyway? Some people associate the word "diet" with deprivation and restrictions. In reality, a "diet" is any style of eating that is either habitual or prescribed. Contrary to popular belief, a healthy diet can taste good and be very satisfying.

Three key factors can turn a "diet" into a "lifestyle." First, you need to **enjoy** what you are eating. Otherwise, you can be certain these changes won't last for a lifetime. Second, the diet needs **flexibility**. People's lives are often unpredictable and busy, so a style of eating that can be easily adapted to your lifestyle is essential. Finally and most importantly, a good diet is one that **promotes health**. Whether it's eating more fruits and vegetables, limiting fat, increasing dietary fiber, reducing portion sizes, or all of these goals, the

result is the promotion of better health. As an added benefit, the characteristics of a healthful diet often result in a more healthful weight.

The Food Guide Pyramid is a key tool in guiding you to eat a healthful diet, and the eating plan is based upon this tool. Each food group provides some, but not all, of the nutrients you need. Foods from one group cannot replace another, and the food groups are equally important. You need to eat from all five tiers of the pyramid for good health.

The foundation of the diet begins with the Bread, Cereal, Rice, and Pasta Group. These foods. when minimally processed, are naturally low in fat and are rich in complex carbohydrates, B vitamins, and fiber. They are often fortified with important minerals such as iron and zinc.

Foods in the Vegetable Group provide you with vitamin A, vitamin C, folate, iron, and magnesium. These foods are also significant sources of fiber and phytochemicals, or plant nutrients.

Foods in the Fruit Group are similar to vegetables because they are wonderful sources of vitamin A, vitamin C, fiber, potassium, and phytochemicals.

The Milk, Yogurt, and Cheese Group provides significant sources of calcium, protein, vitamin D, and phosphorus. Most Americans fail to get adequate amounts of calcium in their daily diets. Choose reduced-fat dairy foods. They contain fewer calories and fat but are calcium-rich.

Foods in the Meat, Poultry, Fish, Beans, and Nuts Group supply protein, iron, zinc, and vitamin B-12. Choose lean cuts of beef and pork to cut fat and calories from this group.

The Fats, Oils, and Sweets Group should enhance the flavor of foods from the lower half of the pyramid. Use them sparingly because they contain little nutrition and are often loaded with calories.

How Does the Food Guide Pyramid Compare to the Food Lists?

This book helps you determine how many calories you should eat each day and provides an appropriate number of servings from each food group in your meal plan. The serving sizes in the Food List are based on the Food Guide Pyramid serving recommendations.

Both the pyramid and the eating plans promote a healthful diet by including variety, balance, and moderation.

Variety All foods can fit into a healthful diet. Eating foods from each of the five food groups helps to ensure adequate nutrition and makes eating more interesting for your palate. Even though your plan contains the same number of bread servings daily, it doesn't mean you have to make the same choices from the bread group each day. Mix it up!

Balance Eating within your meal plan helps you eat enough—but not too much. The number of servings in your plan from each food group is balanced for adequate nutrition. Because the Fats, Oils and Sweets Group packs more calories and fewer nutrients per serving than the other groups, there are fewer servings of this group daily.

Moderation Follow "What's a Portion?" (page 13) as a guide to ideal portion size. Many people eat a healthful diet but gain weight because their portion sizes are too large. It's not necessary to purchase a kitchen scale to measure serving sizes. A deck of cards is about the size of a 3-ounce serving of meat. A computer mouse is the size of a small baked potato. Retain these mental images for reference.

QUIZ: Rate Your Fat Intake

Fat has long been labeled the negative nutrient when it comes to heart health and the fight to lose weight. Because fat contains more than twice the calories per gram as do carbohydrate and protein, cutting the fat in your diet will reduce overall calories. Ask yourself the following:

1. **I drink whole or 2% milk.** Y / N
2. **I eat at least 1 ounce of regular cheese at least four days a week.** Y / N
3. **I usually add cream, half-and-half, or regular non-dairy creamer to my coffee or tea.** Y / N
4. **I snack on ice cream, cake, cookies, and chocolate at least three days a week (excluding the reduced-fat and fat-free varities).** Y / N
5. **I use regular salad dressing, mayonnaise, and sour cream at least three days a week.** Y / N
6. **I eat a fast food meal at least once a week.** Y / N
7. **I eat deep-fried food at least twice a week.** Y / N
8. **I use butter or margarine at most meals.** Y / N
9. **I eat less than one fruit and one vegetable each day.** Y / N

Every "yes" answer means you are eating significant sources of fat that may contribute to excess weight and an increased risk of heart disease. Retake this quiz periodically. Every "yes" that becomes "no" should help you inch closer to your weight loss goal and make your heart happier.

Break Those Old Habits

Do you immediately crave a snack when you sit in front of the television? Do you habitually open the pantry door in search of a snack once you get home from school or work? Eating in a whole new way is easier if you break the old habits that helped put on the pounds in the first place. This is called behavior modification. In short, you can't expect change if your behavior stays the same.

Stop and think about why you eat. Do you eat when your stomach growls or when the clock tells you it is time? Unfortunately, physical hunger is not the only reason we eat. Eating in response to outside cues or feelings (aside from hunger) could contribute to overeating. If you learn to recognize some of these patterns, breaking them is easier.

Physical Reasons Fatigue, illness, tension, pain, sleepiness, premenstrual symptoms, and thirst.

Emotional Reasons Happiness, excitement, anxiety, depression, boredom, anger, worry, and the need for nurturing and/or pleasure.

Situational Reasons Parties, restaurants, movie theaters, sporting events, birthdays, family gatherings, funerals, weddings, meetings, solitude, unstructured time, cooking, coming home (from work or school), watching television, cleaning up after a meal, driving in a car, and breaking one's diet.

External Reasons Sight or smell of food, television commercials or billboards advertising food, and grocery shopping.

If you're eating because you **are** truly hungry, go ahead and eat (if healthful food is available). If you're not hungry but want to eat for any of the reasons listed, you might be able to redirect your desire to eat in another way. For example, if you're tired, you could choose to sleep or rest instead of eating. If you're bored, try another activity to relieve your boredom, such as taking a break at work, calling a friend, surfing the Internet, exercising (see Exercise 101, page 180) or whatever else might decrease your boredom. The alternative activity you choose should be active rather than passive, enjoyable, and incompatible with eating!

Try the following tips to change your behaviors to promote weight loss and weight maintenance.

Pay attention while you are eating. Before eating, take a moment to relax your mind and body. Turn off all distractions such as the television. Many people eat "unconsciously," especially when distracted. As a result, they have no idea how much they've eaten (or overeaten). Pay attention to how your body feels while you are eating. Are you still hungry, or are you getting full? It may take thirty minutes for your body to register feelings of satiety.

Learn to identify when you are physically hungry. Some overweight individuals claim they don't know what it is to feel physically hungry. Taking a moment before eating to "tune in" to your body may be helpful in identifying if you are truly hungry and ready to eat. While eating, try taking a break halfway through your meal to allow your brain time to register signals of satiety.

Have your home and work environments support your weight loss efforts. Clear your house and office of unhealthful, high-calorie, tempting foods that won't help you lose weight. Although you may think that you can resist these tempting foods by sheer willpower, sticking to your meal plan will be easier if you don't have to deal with these foods in your environment. Instead, stock your refrigerator and pantry with more fresh fruits and vegetables and low-calorie food items.

Enlist the support of important others. To make these changes in your life, you need the support of people close to you. Encouragement from friends and family is helpful in strengthening your motivation and providing reinforcement for positive behavior changes. The more your friends and family can adopt your more healthful lifestyle changes, the easier it will be to integrate these changes into your life.

Be easy on yourself during your weight loss process. Remember that making the changes needed for permanent weight loss takes practice and hard work. Be patient with yourself and don't expect perfection. If you have a slip and eat something off your plan, you have not blown your diet! All-or-none thinking can hurt your self-esteem and hinder your success.

In addition to accepting yourself when you temporarily fall back into an old habit, reward yourself for the positive changes you make. Reward yourself when you meet a goal; for example, buy a new outfit if you exercise four times this week. Be sure to choose rewards that are reinforcing to you or they will likely not be as effective.

Finally, be kind to yourself by decreasing the amount of stress in your life. Meditation, relaxation procedures, and regular exercise are effective ways to reduce feelings of stress. Treat yourself to a massage—what a great way to reduce stress and reward yourself!

It Helps to Keep Track

Keeping track of your food intake is an important way to increase your awareness of what, when, how much, and why you are eating. Use the Progress Journal on page 186. It's an easy way to track your daily calories and to identify the behaviors you want to change or reward. Use the information in the table on page 12, the Food Lists on page 13, and the nutritional information with each recipe (including the Healthy Eating Plan Exchanges) to calculate calorie amounts. If it's too difficult to write down what you eat immediately after having a meal or snack, make time at the end of the day. Manage your calories like a checking account. If you spend more than your allotted calorie amount one day, try to spend less the next.

one.breakfast and brunch

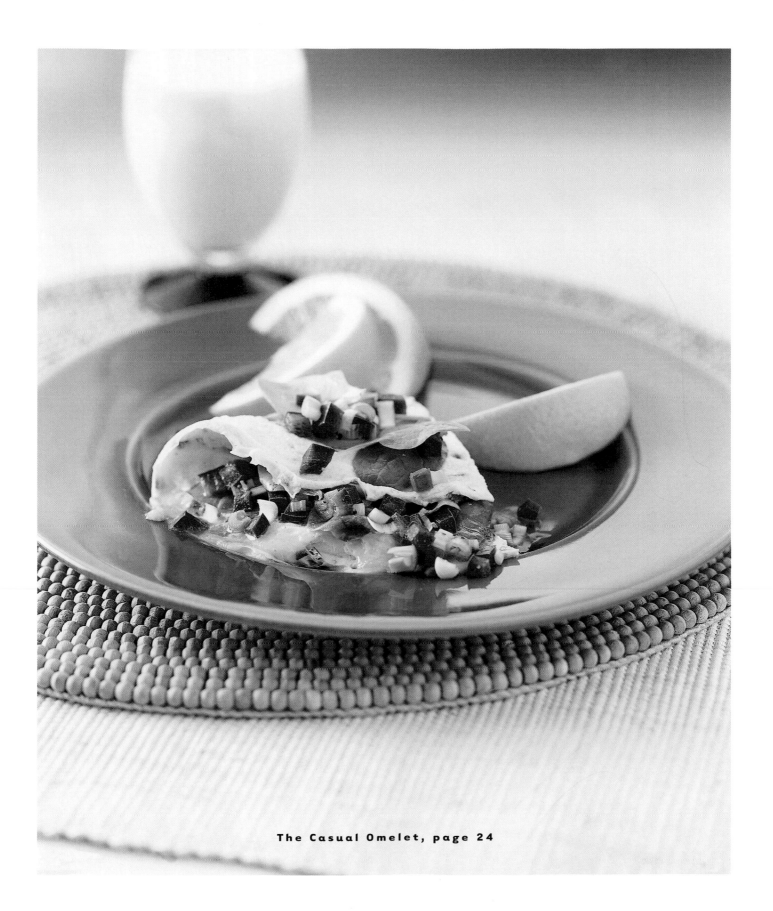

The Casual Omelet, page 24

Breakfast Casserole

Fuel up for a day of biking or hiking with this thyme-flavored ham and potato breakfast casserole. For a little variety, substitute another fresh herb such as basil, oregano, or tarragon.

Exchanges: 1½ Starch, 1 Lean Meat

Nutrition Facts per serving: 180 cal., 4 g total fat (1 g sat. fat), 16 mg chol., 445 mg sodium, 23 g carbo., 1 g fiber, 13 g pro.
Daily Values: 10% vit. A, 26% vit. C, 14% calcium, 16% iron

1	pound tiny new potatoes, cut into ¼-inch slices
⅓	cup thinly sliced leek
	Nonstick cooking spray
¾	cup chopped lower-fat and lower-sodium cooked ham
3	ounces reduced-fat Swiss cheese, cut into small pieces
1¼	cups fat-free milk
1	tablespoon all-purpose flour
¾	cup refrigerated or frozen egg product, thawed
2	teaspoons snipped fresh thyme or ½ teaspoon dried thyme, crushed
¼	teaspoon black pepper

Prep: 25 minutes
Bake: 35 minutes
Makes 6 servings

ONE In a covered large saucepan cook sliced potatoes in a small amount of boiling, lightly salted water about 10 minutes or just until tender, adding the leek the last 5 minutes of cooking. Drain potato mixture. **TWO** Coat a 2-quart rectangular baking dish with cooking spray. Place potato mixture in bottom of the prepared baking dish. Sprinkle with the ham and Swiss cheese. **THREE** In a medium bowl stir the milk into the flour until smooth. Stir in the egg product, thyme, and pepper. Pour the egg mixture over the potato mixture. **FOUR** Bake in a 350° oven for 35 to 40 minutes or until a knife inserted near center comes out clean. Serve immediately.

Eggonomics

Eggs play a crucial role in the success of many recipes. Fortunately it's the binding property found in the fat-free, cholesterol-free egg white that's most often needed. The white, consisting primarily of protein and water, is the main ingredient in most egg substitutes or "egg product." One-fourth cup of egg product equals one whole egg and contains 30 calories, 0 grams fat, and 0 mg cholesterol. Egg product can be used in many recipes that call for whole eggs. Prepare your own substitute by using 2 egg whites for each whole egg. If a recipe requires several eggs or needs a little richness or color, use 2 egg whites and 1 whole egg for every 2 whole eggs.

Cheddar-Polenta Puff

Bold, extra-sharp cheddar cheese mingles with Italian polenta and fluffy egg whites. The result? A satisfying, flavorful breakfast dish that has less than half the fat and cholesterol of a regular cheese soufflé.

Exchanges: ½ Milk, ½ Starch, ½ Lean Meat

Nutrition Facts per serving: 168 cal., 6 g total fat (4 g sat. fat), 69 mg chol., 397 mg sodium, 14 g carbo., 1 g fiber, 13 g pro.
Daily Values: 20% vit. A, 10% vit. C, 21% calcium, 5% iron

4	egg whites
1½	cups fat-free milk
2	tablespoons finely chopped red sweet pepper
1	tablespoon thinly sliced green onion
¼	teaspoon salt
⅛	teaspoon ground red pepper
⅓	cup cornmeal
1	slightly beaten egg yolk
¼	cup shredded extra-sharp cheddar cheese (1 ounce)*
¼	cup grated Parmesan cheese
	Nonstick cooking spray

Prep: 40 minutes
Bake: 25 minutes
Makes 4 servings

ONE Allow egg whites to stand at room temperature for 30 minutes. Meanwhile, in a heavy large saucepan combine milk, sweet pepper, green onion, salt, and ground red pepper. Cook and stir over medium heat until mixture just begins to bubble. Slowly add cornmeal, stirring constantly. Cook and stir about 5 minutes or until mixture begins to thicken. Remove from heat. Stir half of the cornmeal mixture into the egg yolk. Return the yolk mixture to the saucepan. Stir in cheddar and Parmesan cheeses until melted. **TWO** Lightly coat a 1½-quart soufflé dish with cooking spray; set aside. In a large bowl beat egg whites with an electric mixer on medium to high speed until stiff peaks form (tips stand straight). Gently fold about half of the beaten egg whites into the cheese mixture. Gradually pour the cheese mixture over the remaining beaten egg whites, folding to combine. Pour into prepared soufflé dish. **THREE** Bake in a 375° oven about 25 minutes or until a knife inserted in center comes out clean and top is golden brown. Serve immediately.

***Note:** This recipe calls for regular cheddar cheese—not reduced-fat cheddar. The baking time can cause reduced-fat cheese to toughen.*

Baked Brie Strata

Buttery-soft Brie cheese oozes between the layers of tender zucchini and crusty bread for a sure-to-please brunch casserole. Garnish the plates with fresh melon wedges and tiny bunches of grapes.

Exchanges: 1 Milk, 1 Vegetable, ½ Starch, ½ Fat

Nutrition Facts per serving: 198 cal., 8 g total fat (5 g sat. fat), 29 mg chol., 525 mg sodium, 18 g carbo., 1 g fiber, 13 g pro.
Daily Values: 13% vit. A, 13% vit. C, 13% calcium, 9% iron

---

2   small zucchini, cut crosswise into ¼-inch slices (about 2 cups)

    Nonstick cooking spray

6   ½-inch slices crusty sourdough bread

8   ounces Brie cheese, rind removed and cut into ½-inch cubes

2   plum tomatoes, cut lengthwise into ¼-inch slices

6   to 8 cherry tomatoes, halved

1   cup refrigerated or frozen egg product, thawed

⅔   cup evaporated fat-free milk

⅓   cup finely chopped onion

3   tablespoons snipped fresh dill

½   teaspoon salt

⅛   teaspoon black pepper

Prep: 25 minutes
Chill: 4 hours
Bake: 55 minutes
Stand: 10 minutes
Makes 8 servings

ONE In a covered small saucepan cook zucchini in a small amount of boiling, lightly salted water for 2 to 3 minutes or just until tender. Drain zucchini and set aside. **TWO** Meanwhile, coat a 2-quart rectangular baking dish with cooking spray. Arrange bread slices in the bottom of prepared baking dish, cutting as necessary to fit. Sprinkle with half of the cheese. Arrange zucchini and tomatoes on top of cheese. Sprinkle with the remaining cheese. **THREE** In a medium bowl combine egg product, evaporated milk, onion, dill, salt, and pepper. Pour evenly over vegetables and cheese. Press lightly with the back of a spoon to thoroughly moisten ingredients. Cover with plastic wrap and refrigerate for 4 to 24 hours. **FOUR** Remove plastic wrap from strata; cover with foil. Bake in a 325° oven for 30 minutes. Uncover and bake for 25 to 30 minutes more or until a knife inserted near center comes out clean. Let stand for 10 minutes before serving.

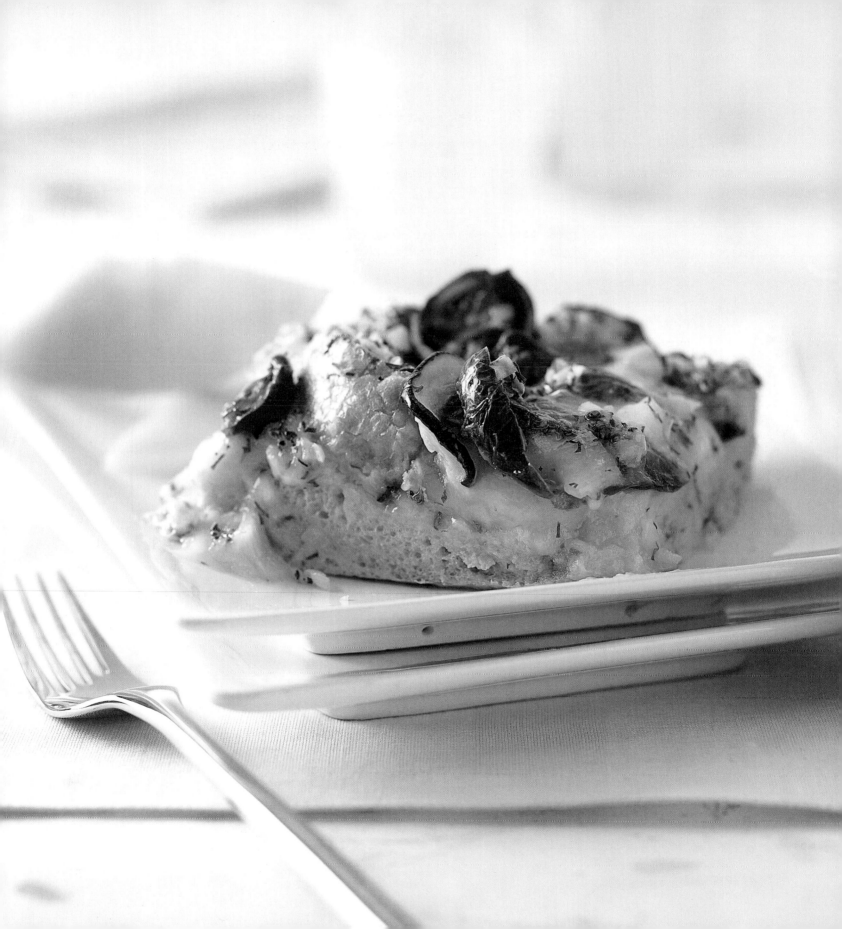

The Casual Omelet

A red pepper relish, loaded with vitamins A and C, adorns these cheese- and spinach-filled omelets. This breakfast classic makes a quick, easy weeknight supper too (see photo, page 19).

Exchanges: ½ Vegetable, 1 Lean Meat

Nutrition Facts per serving: 121 cal., 3 g total fat (2 g sat. fat), 10 mg chol., 380 mg sodium, 7 g carbo., 3 g fiber, 16 g pro.
Daily Values: 51% vit. A, 166% vit. C, 16% calcium, 19% iron

Nonstick cooking spray

1 cup refrigerated or frozen egg product, thawed, or 4 eggs

1 tablespoon snipped fresh chives, Italian flat-leaf parsley, or chervil

Dash salt

Dash ground red pepper

¼ cup shredded reduced-fat sharp cheddar cheese (1 ounce)

1 cup fresh baby spinach leaves or torn spinach

1 recipe Red Pepper Relish

Prep: 10 minutes
Cook: 8 minutes
Makes 2 servings

ONE Coat an 8-inch nonstick skillet with flared sides or a crepe pan with cooking spray. Heat skillet over medium heat. **TWO** In a large bowl combine the egg product, chives, salt, and ground red pepper. Use rotary beater or wire whisk to beat until frothy. Pour into prepared skillet; cook over medium heat. As eggs set, run a spatula around edge of skillet, lifting eggs so uncooked portion flows underneath. **THREE** When eggs are set but still shiny, sprinkle with cheese. Top with ¾ cup of the spinach and 2 tablespoons of the Red Pepper Relish. Fold one side of omelet partially over filling. Top with the remaining spinach and 1 tablespoon of the relish. (Reserve the remaining relish for another use.) Transfer omelet to a warm platter.

Red Pepper Relish

In a small bowl combine ⅔ cup chopped red sweet pepper, 2 tablespoons finely chopped green onion or onion, 1 tablespoon cider vinegar, and ¼ teaspoon black pepper.

Fruited Granola

This cinnamon-scented, berry-packed granola helps you begin any morning with an appetizing crunch. Bowls of this nutritious cereal make great snacks too. If you're out of yogurt, serve this with fat-free milk instead.

Exchanges: ½ Fruit, 1½ Starch, ½ Fat

Nutrition Facts per serving: 216 cal., 4 g total fat (1 g sat. fat), 0 mg chol., 18 mg sodium, 41 g carbo., 6 g fiber, 7 g pro.
Daily Values: 4% vit. A, 6% vit. C, 6% calcium, 14% iron

Nonstick cooking spray

2½ cups regular rolled oats

1 cup whole bran cereal

½ cup toasted wheat germ

¼ cup sliced almonds

½ cup raspberry applesauce

⅓ cup honey

¼ teaspoon ground cinnamon

⅓ cup dried cranberries, blueberries, and/or cherries

Vanilla low-fat yogurt (optional)

Prep: 15 minutes
Bake: 38 minutes
Makes 5 servings

ONE Coat a 15×10×1-inch baking pan with cooking spray; set aside. In a large bowl stir together the rolled oats, bran cereal, wheat germ, and almonds. In a small bowl stir together the applesauce, honey, and cinnamon. Pour the applesauce mixture over cereal mixture; stir until combined. **TWO** Spread the cereal mixture evenly in the prepared baking pan. Bake in a 325° oven for 35 minutes, stirring occasionally. Carefully stir in dried cranberries. Bake for 3 to 5 minutes more or until golden brown. **THREE** Turn out onto a large piece of foil to cool completely. To store, place in an airtight container up to 2 weeks. If desired, serve with vanilla yogurt.

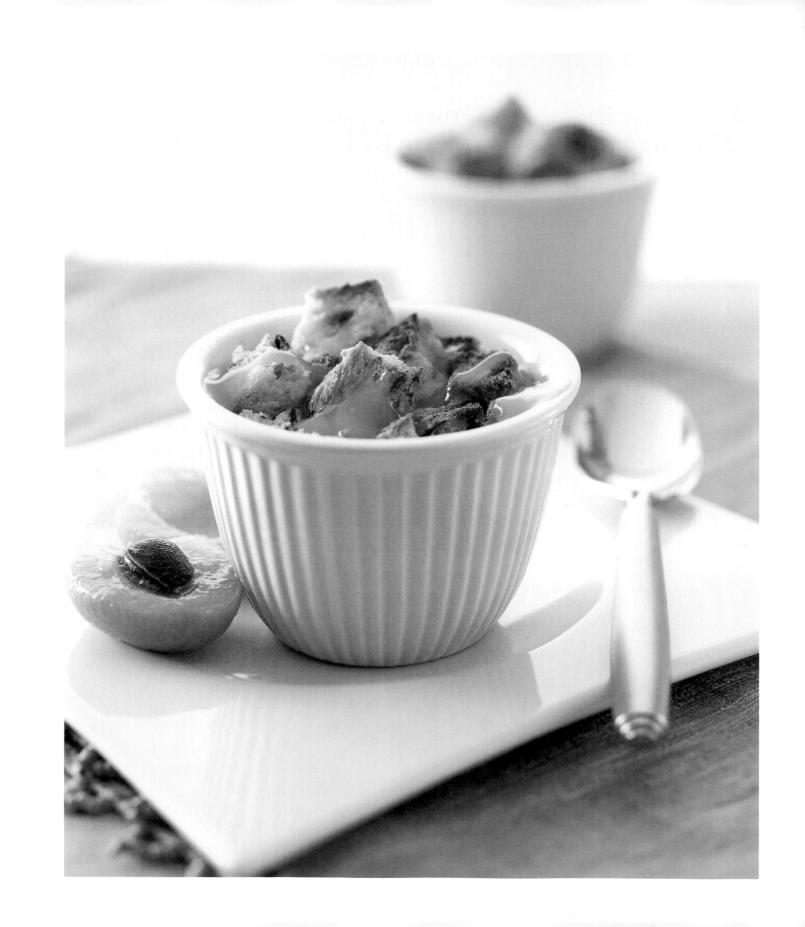

Breakfast Bread Pudding

If you love bread pudding, this is a great way to start the day. Cubes of cinnamon-swirled bread nestle in a custard made with protein-packed egg product and fat-free milk.

Exchanges: ½ Milk, 1½ Starch

Nutrition Facts per serving: 164 cal., 2 g total fat (1 g sat. fat), 1 mg chol., 189 mg sodium, 28 g carbo., 0 g fiber, 8 g pro.
Daily Values: 13% vit. A, 15% vit. C, 9% calcium, 10% iron

6	slices cinnamon-swirl bread or cinnamon-raisin bread
	Nonstick cooking spray
1½	cups fat-free milk
¾	cup refrigerated or frozen egg product, thawed
3	tablespoons sugar
1	teaspoon vanilla
¼	teaspoon ground nutmeg
1	5½-ounce can apricot or peach nectar
2	teaspoons cornstarch

Prep: 25 minutes
Bake: 35 minutes
Stand: 15 minutes
Makes 6 servings

ONE To dry bread, place slices in a single layer on a baking sheet. Bake in a 325° oven for 10 minutes, turning once. Cool on a wire rack. Cut bread into ½-inch cubes (you should have 4 cups). **TWO** Coat six 6-ounce soufflé dishes or custard cups with cooking spray. Divide the bread cubes among the prepared dishes. In a medium bowl combine the milk, egg product, sugar, vanilla, and nutmeg. Use a rotary beater or wire whisk to beat until mixed. Pour the milk mixture evenly over the bread cubes. Press lightly with the back of a spoon to thoroughly moisten bread. **THREE** Place the dishes in a 13×9×2-inch baking pan. Place the baking pan on oven rack. Carefully pour the hottest tap water available into the baking pan around dishes to a depth of 1 inch. **FOUR** Bake in the 325° oven for 35 to 40 minutes or until a knife inserted near center comes out clean. Transfer dishes to a wire rack. Let stand for 15 to 20 minutes. **FIVE** Meanwhile, for sauce, in a small saucepan gradually stir apricot nectar into cornstarch. Cook and stir over medium heat until thickened and bubbly. Reduce heat. Cook and stir for 2 minutes more. Spoon the sauce over puddings.

Breakfast Rice Cereal

Get your day off to a high-fiber, high-energy start with a bowl of hot rice cereal. Sweetened with brown sugar and filled with tiny morsels of dried fruit, it will appeal to the whole family.

Exchanges: ½ Fruit, 1 Starch

Nutrition Facts per serving: 120 cal., 1 g total fat (o g sat. fat), 1 mg chol., 104 mg sodium, 27 g carbo., 1 g fiber, 3 g pro.
Daily Values: 5% vit. A, 1% vit. C, 5% calcium, 1% iron

1½ cups water

⅛ teaspoon salt

1 cup instant brown rice

⅓ cup mixed dried fruit bits

¾ cup fat-free milk

Dash ground nutmeg

4 teaspoons brown sugar

Prep: 10 minutes
Cook: 12 minutes
Makes 4 servings

ONE In a 2-quart saucepan bring the water and salt to boiling. Stir in brown rice; reduce heat. Simmer, covered, for 7 minutes. **TWO** Stir in fruit bits. Simmer, covered, for 5 to 7 minutes more or until rice is tender and liquid is absorbed. Stir in milk and nutmeg. Heat through. Spoon into bowls. Sprinkle each serving with brown sugar.

A Complex Issue

Contrary to popular belief, carbohydrates do not make you fat. Complex carbohydrate sources, such as bread, cereal, pasta, rice, potatoes, and beans, are the foundation of a healthful diet. They are rich in vitamins and minerals and can be excellent sources of fiber as well. The Food Guide Pyramid recommends 6 to 11 servings daily. Eating too many total calories, regardless of the source—carbohydrate, protein, or fat—causes your body to store the extra fuel as fat.

No-Fry French Toast

Crispy, no-fry, hassle-free French toast makes everyone happy. Sweet orange-cinnamon syrup entices breakfast eaters, and the easy, one-batch preparation pleases the cook.

Exchanges: 2 Starch

Nutrition Facts per serving: 171 cal., 3 g total fat (1 g sat. fat), 54 mg chol., 263 mg sodium, 29 g carbo., 0 g fiber, 7 g pro.
Daily Values: 5% vit. A, 26% vit. C, 7% calcium, 8% iron

Nonstick cooking spray

1   slightly beaten egg

1   slightly beaten egg white

3/4   cup fat-free milk

1   teaspoon vanilla

1/8   teaspoon ground cinnamon

8   1/2-inch slices French bread

1/4   teaspoon finely shredded orange peel

1/2   cup orange juice

1   tablespoon honey

1   teaspoon cornstarch

1/8   teaspoon ground cinnamon

1   tablespoon sifted powdered sugar (optional)

Prep: 15 minutes
Bake: 11 minutes
Makes 4 servings

ONE Coat a large baking sheet with cooking spray; set aside. In a pie plate combine the egg, egg white, milk, vanilla, and 1/8 teaspoon cinnamon. Soak the bread slices in egg mixture about 1 minute on each side. Place on the prepared baking sheet. **TWO** Bake in a 450° oven about 6 minutes or until the bread is lightly browned. Turn bread; bake for 5 to 8 minutes more or until golden brown. **THREE** Meanwhile, for orange syrup, in a small saucepan stir together the orange peel, orange juice, honey, cornstarch, and 1/8 teaspoon cinnamon. Cook and stir over medium heat until thickened and bubbly. Reduce heat. Cook and stir 2 minutes more. **FOUR** If desired, sprinkle with powdered sugar and serve with warm orange syrup.

Tropical Coffee Cake

Mango and coconut give this yummy coffee cake an island flair. Yogurt and a small amount of oil keep the cake moist. If you can't find mangoes, substitute nectarines or peaches.

Exchanges: 2 Starch, ½ Fat

Nutrition Facts per serving: 193 cal., 5 g total fat (1 g sat. fat), 27 mg chol., 194 mg sodium, 34 g carbo., 1 g fiber, 4 g pro.
Daily Values: 11% vit. A, 12% vit. C, 5% calcium, 7% iron

1¼ cups all-purpose flour

½ cup sugar

½ teaspoon baking powder

½ teaspoon baking soda

¼ teaspoon salt

¼ teaspoon ground nutmeg

1 beaten egg

⅔ cup plain fat-free yogurt

2 tablespoons cooking oil

½ teaspoon vanilla

1 medium mango, seeded, peeled, and finely chopped (see tip, page 110)

1 tablespoon all-purpose flour

2 tablespoons flaked coconut

Prep: 25 minutes
Bake: 35 minutes
Makes 8 servings

ONE Lightly grease and flour a 9×1½-inch round baking pan; set aside. In a large bowl stir together the 1¼ cups flour, the sugar, baking powder, baking soda, salt, and nutmeg. Make a well in the center of the flour mixture; set aside. **TWO** In a small bowl stir together the egg, yogurt, oil, and vanilla. Add all at once to the flour mixture. Stir just until moistened (batter should be slightly lumpy). In a small bowl toss chopped mango with the 1 tablespoon flour; gently fold into batter. Spread the batter into the prepared baking pan. Sprinkle with coconut. **THREE** Bake in a 350° oven about 35 minutes or until a wooden toothpick inserted near center comes out clean. Serve warm.

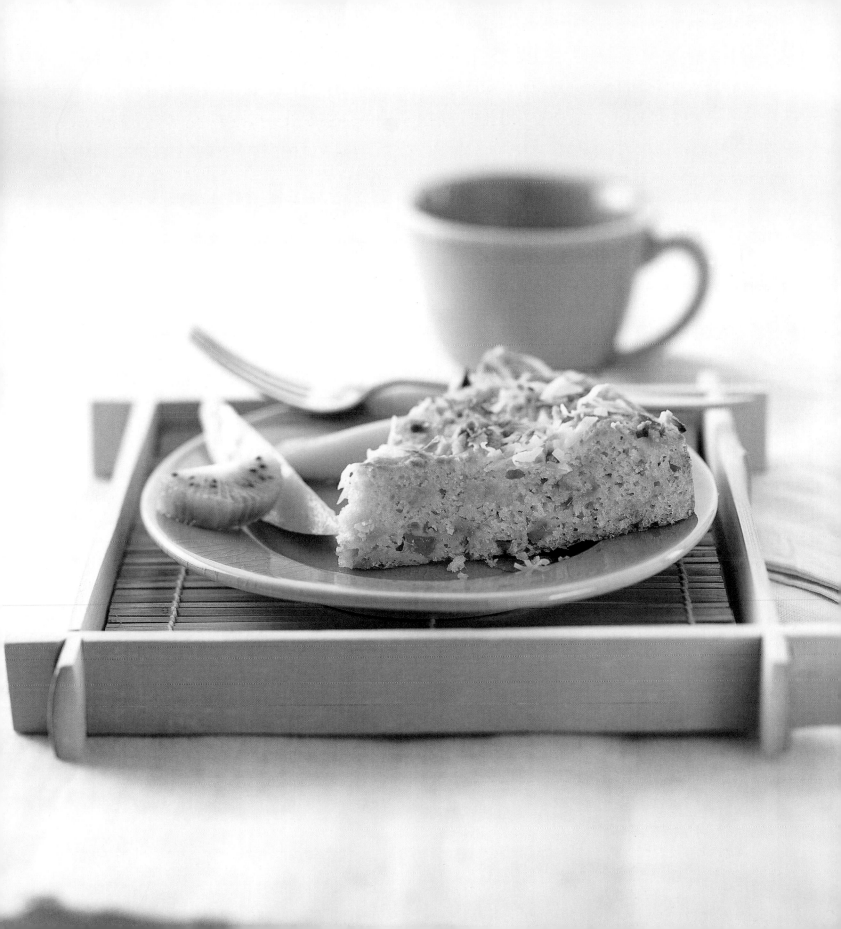

Blueberry Breakfast Scones

Bake a batch of these scrumptious scones for a light summer breakfast or anytime snack. A little orange peel and a drizzle of tangy orange icing boosts the fruity flavor.

Exchanges: 2 Starch, 1 Fat

Nutrition Facts per serving: 194 cal., 5 g total fat (1 g sat. fat), 1 mg chol., 273 mg sodium, 34 g carbo., 1 g fiber, 4 g pro.
Daily Values: 7% vit. A, 6% vit. C, 10% calcium, 9% iron

Nonstick cooking spray

2 cups all-purpose flour

¼ cup sugar

1 tablespoon baking powder

1 tablespoon finely shredded orange peel

¼ teaspoon baking soda

¼ teaspoon salt

¼ cup margarine or butter

½ cup buttermilk or sour fat-free milk*

¼ cup refrigerated or frozen egg product, thawed

1 teaspoon vanilla

1 cup fresh blueberries or frozen blueberries, thawed and drained

1 recipe Orange Powdered Sugar Icing

Prep: 20 minutes
Bake: 15 minutes
Makes 10 scones

ONE Coat a baking sheet with cooking spray; set aside. In a large bowl stir together flour, sugar, baking powder, orange peel, baking soda, and salt. Using a pastry blender, cut in margarine until mixture resembles coarse crumbs. Make a well in center of flour mixture. In a small bowl stir together buttermilk, egg product, and vanilla. Add all at once to the flour mixture. Stir with a fork just until moistened. Gently stir in blueberries. **TWO** Turn dough out onto a lightly floured surface. Quickly knead dough by gently folding and pressing dough for 12 to 15 strokes or until nearly smooth. Working on the prepared baking sheet, pat dough into a 7-inch circle. Cut into 10 wedges. **THREE** Bake in a 400° oven for 15 to 20 minutes or until golden brown. Remove from baking sheet; cool on a wire rack while preparing Orange Powdered Sugar Icing. Drizzle the icing over tops of scones. Serve warm.

Orange Powdered Sugar Icing:

In a bowl combine ¾ cup sifted powdered sugar and ¼ teaspoon finely shredded orange peel. Stir in enough orange juice or fat-free milk (3 to 4 teaspoons) to make an icing of drizzling consistency.

*Note: *To make sour milk, place 1½ teaspoons lemon juice or vinegar in a glass measure. Add fat-free milk to equal ½ cup.*

Super Soy Smoothies
Soy milk is readily available in the dairy section of most grocery stores. Because soy milk contains less calcium than cow milk, some brands are fortified with this important mineral. If calcium is a concern, choose a fortified brand.

Exchanges: 1½ Fruit

Nutrition Facts per serving: 96 cal., 1 g total fat (0 g sat. fat), 0 mg chol., 6 mg sodium, 21 g carbo., 2 g fiber, 2 g pro.
Daily Values: 3% vit. A, 39% vit. C, 1% calcium, 3% iron

½ of a 16-ounce package frozen unsweetened peach slices (about 2 cups)

1 medium banana, cut up

¾ cup vanilla soy milk or plain soy milk

¼ cup frozen orange-pineapple juice concentrate, thawed

1 cup ice cubes

Prep: 10 minutes
Makes 4 (¾-cup) servings

ONE Set aside 4 peach slices for garnish. In a blender container combine the remaining peaches, the banana, soy milk, and juice concentrate. Cover and blend until smooth. Gradually add the ice cubes through the hole in the blender lid, blending until smooth after each addition. **TWO** To serve, pour mixture into 4 chilled glasses. Garnish each glass with a peach slice.

The Soy Sensation

Soy products such as soy milk, green soybeans, tofu, and tempeh are currently being promoted as the ticket to good health. The most well-documented healthful effect of soy is its ability to lower cholesterol levels. Eating 25 grams of soy protein per day can reduce cholesterol levels by up to 10 percent. Stay tuned for more good news in the future as researchers continue to investigate the role of soy in preventing cancer and helping ease the symptoms of menopause.

two.starters and snacks

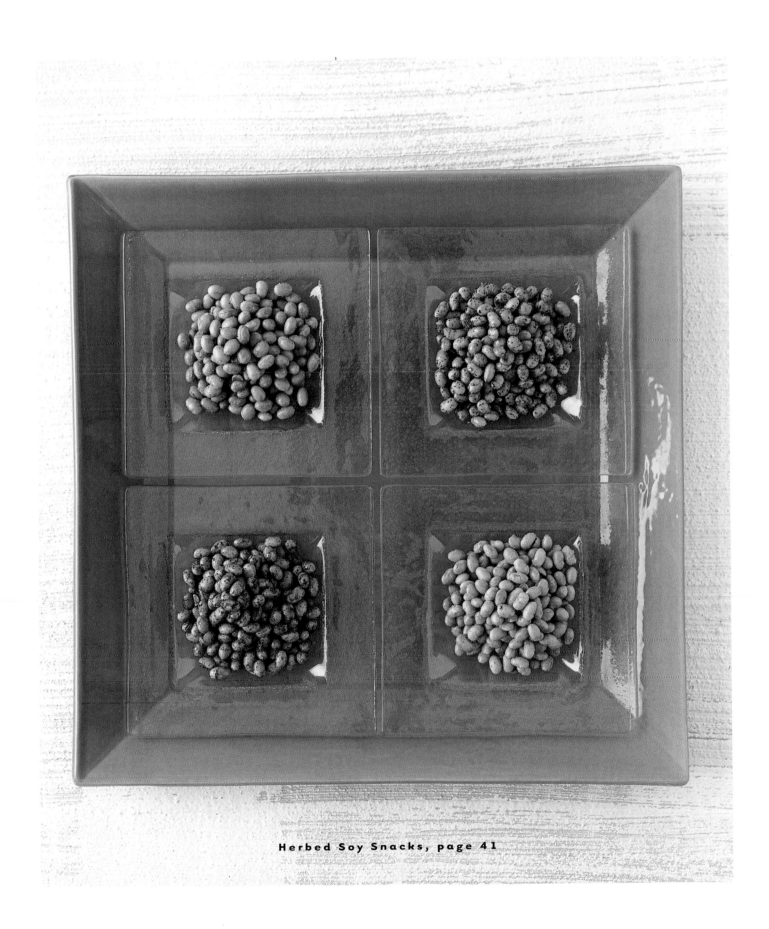

Herbed Soy Snacks, page 41

Incredible Quesadillas

Capture a South-of-the-border attitude with these wickedly rich, flavor-packed snacks. Stuffed with reduced-fat sausage and cheese, they have all the zip of traditional quesadillas but a lot fewer calories.

Exchanges: ½ Starch, ½ Lean Meat

Nutrition Facts per serving: 104 cal., 2 g total fat (1 g sat. fat), 8 mg chol., 362 mg sodium, 17 g carbo., 2 g fiber, 5 g pro.
Daily Values: 2% vit. A, 1% vit. C, 4% calcium, 2% iron

½ cup shredded reduced-fat taco cheese

4 8-inch fat-free flour tortillas

4 reduced-fat brown-and-serve sausage links, cooked and coarsely chopped

1 small red onion, sliced and separated into rings

2 tablespoons finely snipped fresh cilantro

2 tablespoons well-drained pineapple salsa or regular salsa

½ cup pineapple salsa or regular salsa

Prep: 20 minutes
Cook: 12 minutes
Makes 8 appetizer servings

ONE Preheat a waffle baker to a medium-high heat setting.* Sprinkle 2 tablespoons of the cheese over half of each tortilla. Top with sausage, onion, cilantro, and the 2 tablespoons salsa. Fold tortillas in half, pressing gently. **TWO** Place a quesadilla on preheated waffle baker. Close lid, pressing slightly. Bake for 3 to 6 minutes or until tortilla is lightly browned and cheese is melted. Remove from waffle baker. Repeat with the remaining quesadillas. Cut quesadillas in half. Serve the quesadilla pieces with the ½ cup salsa.

***Note:** Or, use a large nonstick skillet to cook each quesadilla over medium heat for 3 to 4 minutes or until golden brown. Using a spatula, turn quesadilla. Cook for 2 to 3 minutes more or until golden brown.*

Artichoke-Feta Tortilla Wraps

Three cheeses mingle with roasted sweet peppers and artichoke hearts in these tortilla-wrapped treats. They're perfect appetizers for a casual gathering of friends.

Exchanges: ½ Vegetable, ½ Starch, ½ Fat

Nutrition Facts per serving: 75 cal., 4 g total fat (2 g sat. fat), 8 mg chol., 177 mg sodium, 8 g carbo., 1 g fiber, 3 g pro.
Daily Values: 2% vit. A, 26% vit. C, 7% calcium, 4% iron

Nonstick cooking spray

1   14-ounce can artichoke hearts, drained and finely chopped

½   of an 8-ounce tub reduced-fat cream cheese (Neufchâtel), about ½ cup

3   green onions, thinly sliced

⅓   cup grated Parmesan or Romano cheese

¼   cup crumbled feta cheese

3   tablespoons reduced-fat pesto

8   8-inch spinach, tomato, or regular flour tortillas

1   7-ounce jar roasted red sweet peppers, drained and cut into strips

1   recipe Yogurt-Chive Sauce

Prep: 15 minutes
Bake: 15 minutes
Makes 24 appetizer servings

ONE Coat a 3-quart rectangular baking dish with cooking spray; set aside. For filling, in a large bowl stir together the artichoke hearts, cream cheese, green onions, Parmesan cheese, feta cheese, and pesto. **TWO** Place about ¼ cup filling on each tortilla. Top with red pepper strips; roll up. Arrange tortilla rolls in the prepared baking dish. If desired, lightly coat tortilla rolls with additional cooking spray. Bake, uncovered, in a 350° oven about 15 minutes or until heated through. **THREE** Cut each tortilla roll into thirds and arrange on a serving platter. Serve with Yogurt-Chive Sauce.

Yogurt-Chive Sauce:
In a small bowl stir together one 8-ounce carton plain fat-free yogurt and 1 tablespoon snipped fresh chives. Chill until serving time.

A Little Goes a Long Way
For the true cheese lover, life without cheese is the ultimate sacrifice. Eliminating cheese from the menu, even when trying to lose weight, means missing out on a rich source of calcium, protein, vitamin D, and phosphorus. To include cheese in your meals and keep fat in check, choose strongly flavored varieties such as Parmesan, Romano, feta, Asiago, or sharp cheddar—you'll need smaller amounts to get a rich, cheesy flavor.

Vegetable Spring Rolls

Translucent rice papers encase a mixture of zestfully spiced daikon, jalapeño peppers, carrots, and cucumbers. Look for daikon and the rice papers in the specialty produce section of your supermarket or at an Asian food store.

Exchanges: 1 Vegetable

Nutrition Facts per serving: 31 cal., 0 g total fat (0 g sat. fat), 0 mg chol., 48 mg sodium, 7 g carbo., 0 g fiber, 0 g pro.
Daily Values: 14% vit. A, 7% vit. C, 1% iron

½ cup shredded daikon (Oriental white radish) or radishes

2 green onions, thinly sliced

2 tablespoons rice vinegar

1 small fresh jalapeño or serrano pepper, seeded and finely chopped (see tip, page 153)

1 teaspoon sugar

½ teaspoon toasted sesame oil

½ cup shredded carrot

½ cup bite-size cucumber strips

2 tablespoons snipped fresh cilantro

1 tablespoon reduced-sodium soy sauce

1 cup warm water

6 8½-inch rice papers

1½ cups shredded Boston or curly leaf lettuce

Prep: 30 minutes
Chill: 2 hours
Makes 12 appetizer servings

ONE In a small bowl combine daikon, green onions, vinegar, jalapeño pepper, sugar, and sesame oil. In another bowl combine shredded carrot, cucumber, cilantro, and soy sauce. Cover both mixtures; refrigerate for 2 to 24 hours, stirring once. Drain both mixtures. **TWO** Pour the warm water into a pie plate. Carefully dip rice papers into water, one at a time. Place papers, not touching, on clean, dry kitchen towels. Let soften for a few minutes until pliable. **THREE** Place ¼ cup shredded lettuce on each rice paper, near one edge. Place about 1 rounded tablespoon of each vegetable mixture on the lettuce. Fold in the ends. Beginning at that edge, tightly roll up the filled rice paper. Place, seam side down, on a plate. Cover with a damp towel. Repeat with the remaining fillings and papers. Cover; refrigerate up to 2 hours. **FOUR** To serve, cut each roll in half crosswise on a diagonal to make 12 pieces.

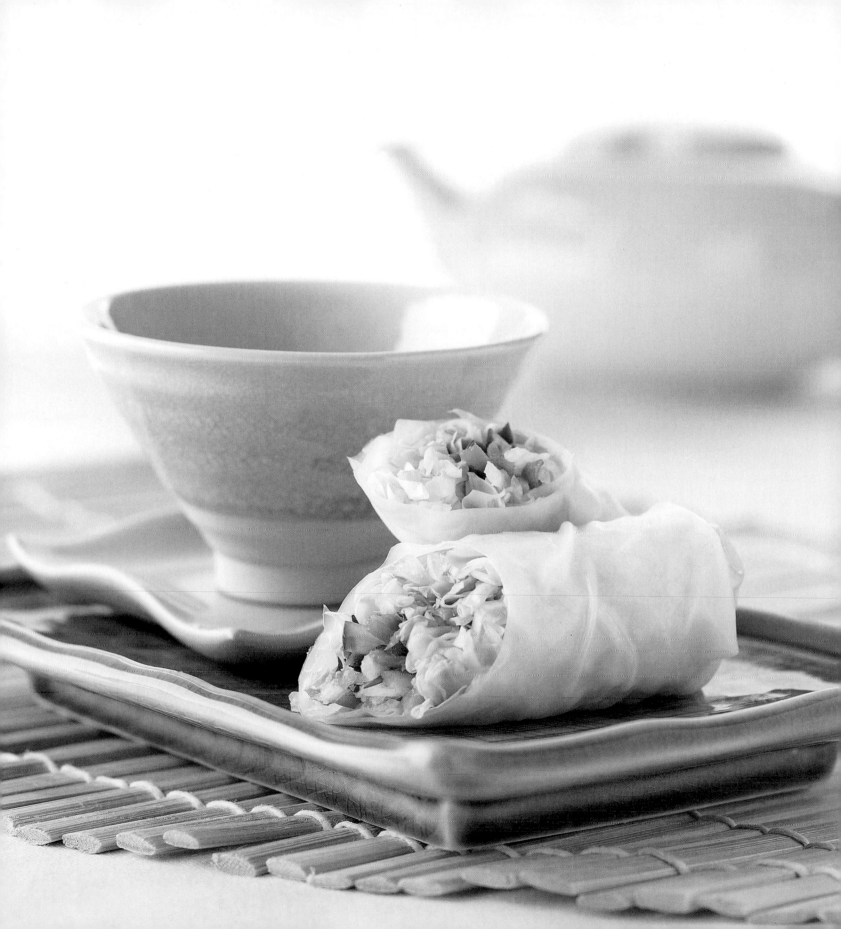

Energy Bars

These sweet, moist treats provide a surprise protein punch from pinto beans. They'll not only help you get up and go, they'll also keep you going. Take a frozen bar to the office to revive waning energy during the day.

Exchanges: ½ Fruit, 1 Starch, ½ Fat

Nutrition Facts per serving: 137 cal., 5 g total fat (1 g sat. fat), 9 mg chol., 90 mg sodium, 24 g carbo., 2 g fiber, 2 g pro.
Daily Values: 1% calcium, 5% iron

Nonstick cooking spray

1²/3 cups low-fat granola

1 cup flaked coconut

1 cup chopped pitted dates

²/3 cup packed light brown sugar

½ cup whole wheat pastry flour

1 teaspoon ground cinnamon

1 15-ounce can pinto or Great Northern beans, rinsed, well drained, and coarsely chopped

½ cup dark raisins

½ cup chopped walnuts or almonds

½ cup honey

3 tablespoons margarine or butter, melted

2 tablespoons cooking oil

1 teaspoon vanilla

⅛ teaspoon salt

Prep: 20 minutes
Bake: 40 minutes
Makes 30 bars

ONE Line a 13×9×2-inch baking pan with foil; lightly coat the foil with cooking spray. Set aside. **TWO** In a large bowl combine the granola, coconut, dates, brown sugar, flour, and cinnamon. Stir in beans, raisins, and nuts. In a small bowl combine honey, margarine, oil, vanilla, and salt. Add to cereal mixture; stir until combined. Spread evenly in the prepared baking pan. **THREE** Bake in a 350° oven for 40 to 45 minutes or until the edges are lightly browned and the center is firm to touch. Cool completely. Use foil to lift bars out of pan; cut into pieces. If desired, wrap bars in foil and freeze for up to 3 months.

Herbed Soy Snacks

Choose your seasoning to perk up dry roasted soybeans. This crunchy snack provides healthful phytonutrients for your diet. Look for dry roasted soy beans in your local supermarket or health food store (see photo, page 35).

Exchanges: ½ Lean Meat, ½ Fat

Nutrition Facts per serving: 75 cal., 3 g total fat (1 g sat. fat), 0 mg chol., 27 mg sodium, 4 g carbo., 2 g fiber, 7 g pro.
Daily Values: 1% vit. A, 3% calcium, 5% iron

8	ounces dry roasted soybeans (2 cups)
1½	teaspoons dried thyme, crushed
¼	teaspoon garlic salt
⅛	to ¼ teaspoon ground red pepper

Prep: 5 minutes
Bake: 5 minutes
Makes 16 (2-tablespoon) servings

ONE Spread roasted soybeans in an even layer in a 15×10×1-inch baking pan. In a small bowl combine thyme, garlic salt, and red pepper. Sprinkle the soybeans with the thyme mixture. Bake in a 350° oven about 5 minutes or just until heated through, shaking pan once. Cool completely. **TWO** To store, place in an airtight container at room temperature for up to 1 week. To use, eat plain, toss in soups or salads, sprinkle on baked potatoes, or mix with popcorn or other party mixes.

Curried Soy Snacks:
Prepare Herbed Soy Snacks as directed, except combine 1 teaspoon curry powder and ¼ teaspoon salt; sprinkle over soybeans before baking. Omit thyme, garlic salt, and ground red pepper.

Sweet Chili Soy Snacks:
Prepare Herbed Soy Snacks as directed, except increase garlic salt to ½ teaspoon and combine with 2 teaspoons brown sugar and 1½ teaspoons chili powder; sprinkle over soybeans before baking. Omit thyme and ground red pepper.

Mustard Soy Snacks:
Prepare Herbed Soy Snacks as directed, except combine 1½ teaspoons paprika, ½ teaspoon dry mustard, and ¼ teaspoon salt; sprinkle over soybeans before baking. Omit thyme, garlic salt, and ground red pepper.

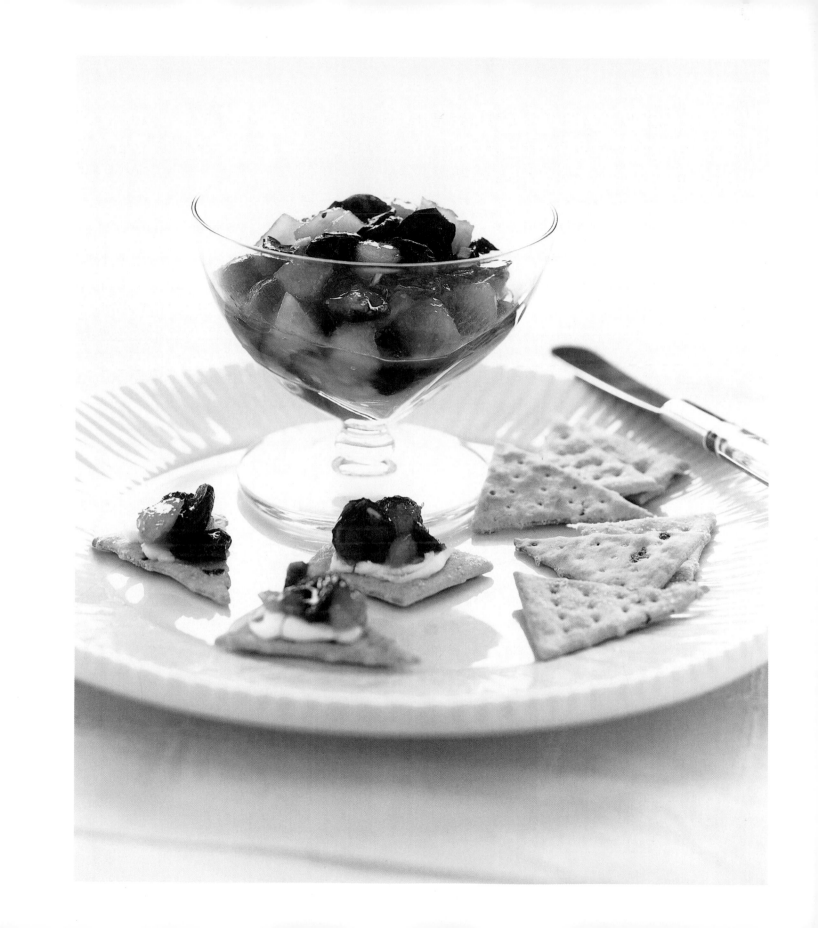

Dried Cranberry Chutney Appetizers

Just add four ingredients to purchased chutney and make taste buds tingle with delight. Serve a spoonful on pear wedges for another variation of this fat-free snack.

Exchanges: ½ Fruit

Nutrition Facts per serving: 37 cal., 0 g total fat (0 g sat. fat), 0 mg chol., 2 mg sodium, 9 g carbo., 0 g fiber, 0 g pro.
Daily Values: 2% vit. A

½	cup dried cranberries
¼	cup water
2	tablespoons sugar
1	tablespoon finely chopped fresh ginger
¾	cup mango chutney
	Fat-free cream cheese
	Apple slices
	Crackers or toasted baguette slices

Prep: 20 minutes
Chill: 2 hours
Makes 22 (1-tablespoon) servings

ONE In a small saucepan combine dried cranberries, water, sugar, and ginger. Bring to boiling. Cover and remove from heat. Let stand for 15 minutes. **TWO** Snip any large pieces of mango chutney. Stir the chutney into cranberry mixture. Cover and refrigerate for at least 2 hours. **THREE** Serve the cranberry chutney with fat-free cream cheese, apple slices, and crackers or baguette slices.

Are You an Apple or a Pear?

Are you shaped like an apple or a pear? Body shapes differ, depending on where fat is stored. Where your body stores fat is a clue to your general health. Accumulation of body fat in the stomach area and waistline, giving an apple shape, might put a person at risk for heart disease, high blood pressure, and diabetes. (The waist measurement should not exceed 40 inches for men and 35 inches for women.) Fat stored below the waist in the hips, buttocks, and thighs—the pear shape—might not be as risky for your overall health.

Mediterranean Walnut Spread

Aromatic basil and tangy lemon juice complement the hearty flavor of ground garbanzo beans and walnuts in this simple spread. Add the remaining garbanzo beans to a salad, soup, or stew.

Exchanges: ½ Fat

Nutrition Facts per serving: 34 cal., 3 g total fat (0 g sat. fat), 0 mg chol., 25 mg sodium, 1 g carbo., 0 g fiber, 1 g pro.

Daily Values: 1% iron

---

1   cup canned garbanzo beans (about ½ of a 15-ounce can)

½   cup chopped walnuts

½   cup lightly packed fresh basil

2   tablespoons olive oil

2   to 3 teaspoons lemon juice

⅛   teaspoon salt

⅛   teaspoon black pepper

Toasted thin baguette slices or pita bread slices

Start to Finish: 15 minutes
Makes 20 (1-tablespoon) servings

ONE Drain garbanzo beans, reserving the liquid. In a blender container or food processor bowl combine beans and 2 tablespoons of the reserved liquid. Add walnuts, basil, olive oil, lemon juice, salt, and pepper. Cover and blend or process until nearly smooth. (Scrape down sides and add additional reserved liquid if the mixture is stiff.)

TWO Serve the spread on toasted baguette or pita bread slices. To store, place in an airtight container in the refrigerator for up to 5 days.

Crispy, Toasty Dippers

Next time you need a low-calorie "scoop" for your favorite dip or salsa, try one of these crispy dippers.

Pita Wedges: Split pita bread rounds in half. Cut each half into 6 wedges. Place, cut sides up, on an ungreased baking sheet. Bake in a 375° oven for 7 to 9 minutes or until lightly browned.

Baguette Slices: Cut an 8-ounce baguette into ½-inch slices. Place slices on an ungreased baking sheet. Bake in a 425° oven about 5 minutes or until light brown, turning once.

Tortilla Crisps: Cut 6-inch flour or corn tortillas into 6 wedges each. Place wedges in a single layer on an ungreased baking sheet. Bake in a 350° oven for 8 to 10 minutes or until crisp.

Strawberries with Lime Dipping Sauce

Juicy, sweet strawberries dipped in a tangy lime sauce provide half of your daily vitamin C requirement. To keep berries fresh, wait until just before serving to clean them.

Exchanges: 1 Fruit

Nutrition Facts per serving: 60 cal., 2 g total fat (1 g sat. fat), 4 mg chol., 33 mg sodium, 9 g carbo., 1 g fiber, 2 g pro.
Daily Values: 3% vit. A, 54% vit. C, 3% calcium, 1% iron

1   8-ounce carton light or fat-free dairy sour cream

2   tablespoons powdered sugar

2   teaspoons finely shredded lime peel

1   tablespoon lime juice

3   cups small strawberries

Prep: 10 minutes
Makes 8 servings

ONE For lime dipping sauce, in a small bowl stir together sour cream, powdered sugar, lime peel, and lime juice; set aside. **TWO** Wash strawberries, but do not remove stems. Drain on several layers of paper towels. Serve the strawberries with the lime dipping sauce.

Fruit Kabobs

For a refreshing treat on hot summer days, dunk these citrus-marinated fruit kabobs in an orange-scented vanilla yogurt sauce. To save time, purchase cut-up fresh fruit from the salad bar or produce section in your supermarket.

Exchanges: 1½ Fruit

Nutrition Facts per serving: 91 cal., 1 g total fat (0 g sat. fat), 2 mg chol., 20 mg sodium, 21 g carbo., 1 g fiber, 2 g pro.
Daily Values: 6% vit. A, 78% vit. C, 4% calcium, 2% iron

³/₄   cup papaya chunks

³/₄   cup honeydew melon or
      cantaloupe chunks

³/₄   cup small strawberries

³/₄   cup pineapple chunks

2   small bananas, cut into 1-inch
    slices

1   cup orange juice

¼   cup lime juice

1   8-ounce carton vanilla low-fat or
    fat-free yogurt

2   tablespoons frozen orange juice
    concentrate, thawed

Prep: 20 minutes
Marinate: 30 minutes
Makes 8 servings

ONE On eight 6-inch or four 10-inch skewers alternately thread the papaya, honeydew melon, strawberries, pineapple, and bananas. Place kabobs in a shallow glass dish. Combine orange juice and lime juice; pour evenly over kabobs. Cover and chill in the refrigerator for 30 to 60 minutes, turning occasionally. **TWO** Meanwhile, for dip, in a small bowl stir together the yogurt and orange juice concentrate. Cover and refrigerate until ready to serve. **THREE** To serve, arrange the kabobs on a serving platter; discard the juice mixture. Serve the kabobs with the dip.

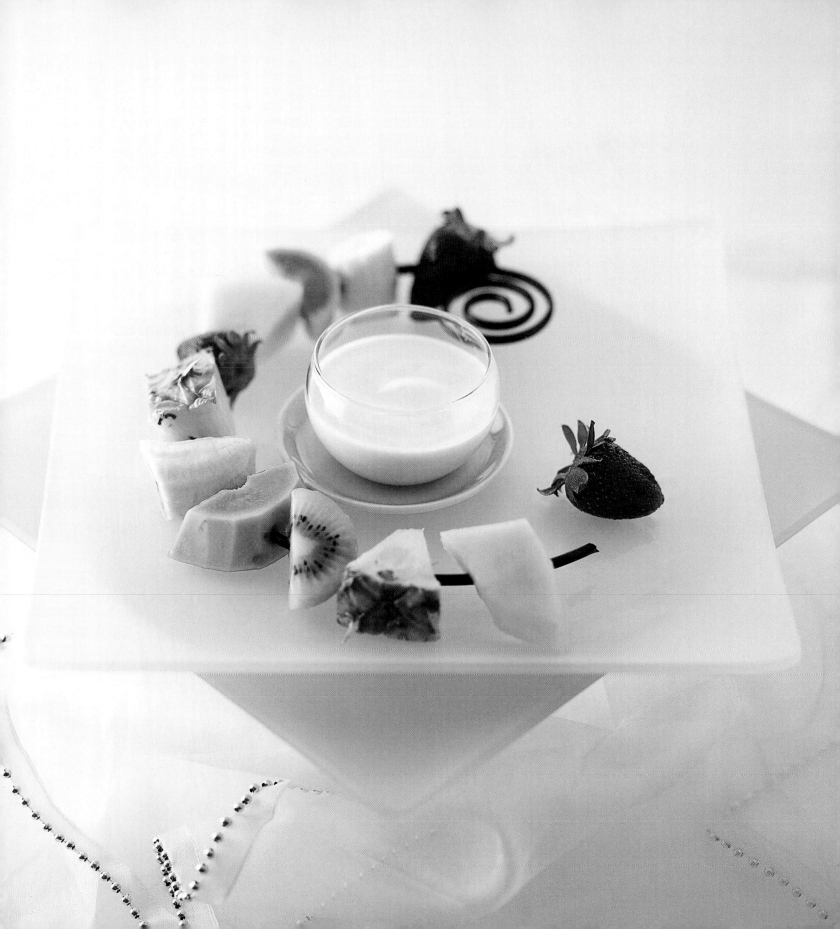

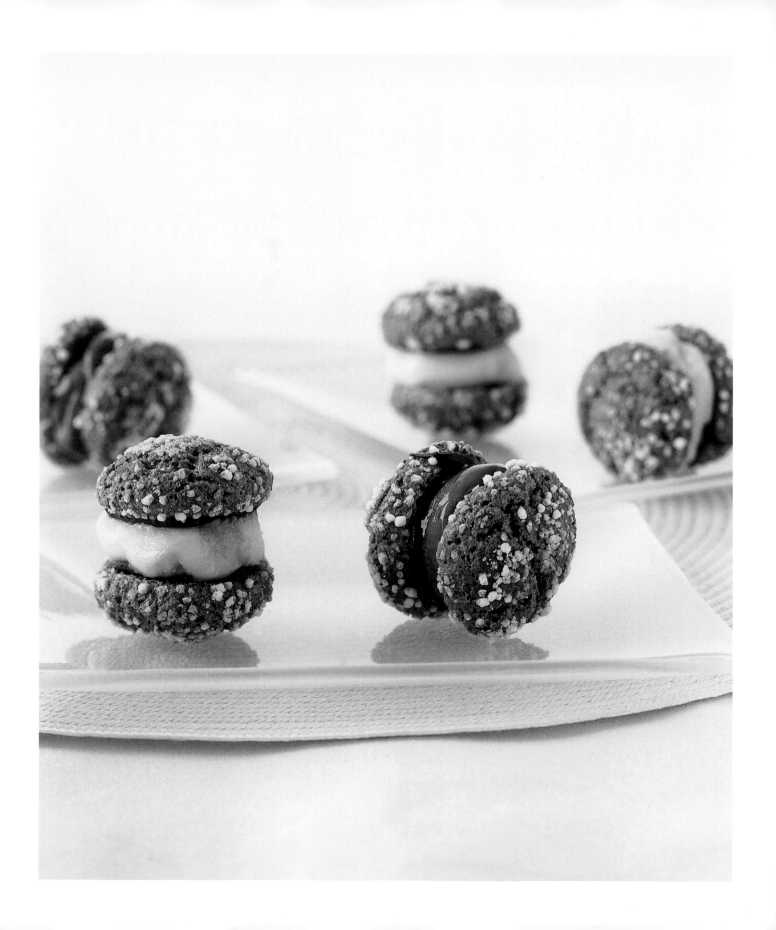

Yo-Yos

Nibble on these bite-size snacks without guilt. To make them, spread amaretti cookies with a little melted chocolate and put a small scoop of your favorite fruit-flavored sorbet between two of the cookies.

Exchanges: 1 Starch, ½ Fat

Nutrition Facts per serving: 71 cal., 2 g total fat (0 g sat. fat), 6 mg chol., 7 mg sodium, 12 g carbo., 0 g fiber, 1 g pro.
Daily Values: 1% vit. A, 2% calcium, 4% iron

¼ cup semisweet chocolate pieces

¼ teaspoon shortening

24 amaretti cookies (4.6 ounces total) or vanilla wafers

⅓ cup mango, orange, lemon, or raspberry sorbet

Prep: 30 minutes
Freeze: 1 hour
Makes 6 servings

ONE In a heavy small saucepan heat chocolate pieces and shortening over low heat just until melted. Cool slightly. Using a narrow metal spatula, spread about 1 teaspoon of the chocolate mixture on the flat sides of half the cookies. Place coated cookies, chocolate sides up, on a wire rack until the chocolate mixture is set. **TWO** Using a melon baller, place a small scoop of sorbet (about 1 rounded teaspoon) on the chocolate side of each coated cookie. Dip the melon baller into water between scoops to make the scoops come out neatly. Top sorbet with an uncoated cookie to make a sandwich. Cover and freeze for 1 to 4 hours before serving.

Lose a Little, Gain a Lot

Need more incentive for winning the battle of the bulge? Here's some encouraging news. Most of the health benefits of weight loss can be achieved with a modest drop in pounds. A decrease in body weight of only 5 to 10 percent can substantially improve blood pressure, lower cholesterol levels, and reduce the odds of developing diabetes. For example, a 200-pound individual who loses as little as 10 pounds could experience these benefits.

three.salads

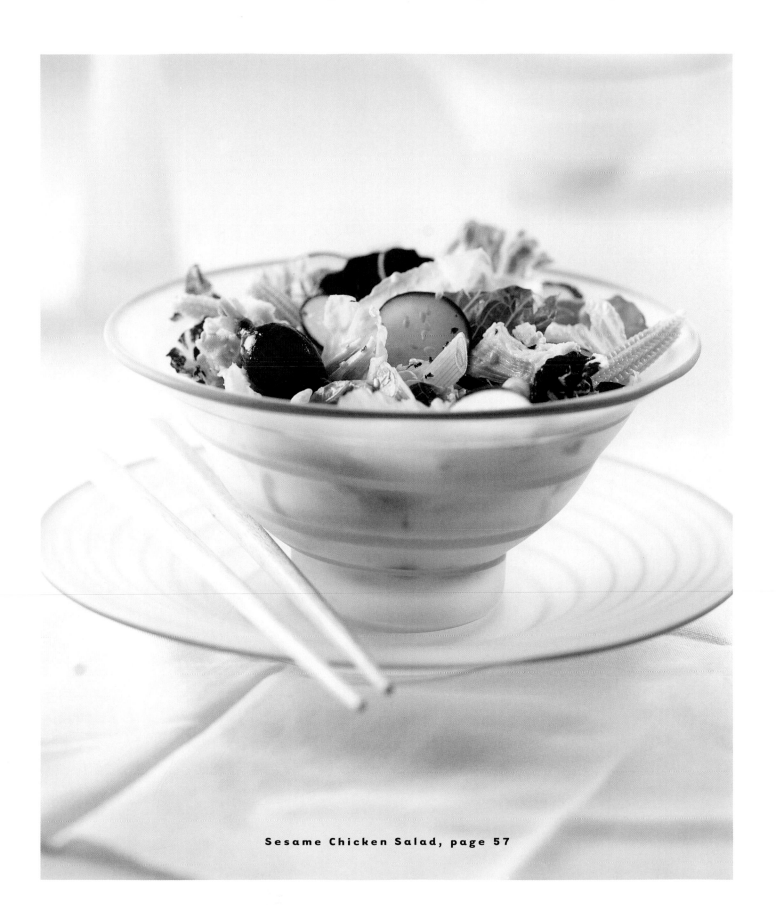

Sesame Chicken Salad, page 57

Spicy Steak and Ranch Salad

Cajun-seasoned steak teams with crunchy French-fried onions and cool, crisp greens for a main-dish salad that can satisfy even the heartiest appetite.

Exchanges: 2 Vegetable, 2 Lean Meat, 1 Fat

Nutrition Facts per serving: 310 cal., 13 g total fat (4 g sat. fat), 76 mg chol., 557 mg sodium, 16 g carbo., 3 g fiber, 28 g pro.
Daily Values: 126% vit. A, 40% vit. C, 5% calcium, 28% iron

½ cup French-fried onions

1   pound boneless beef top sirloin steak, cut 1 inch thick

1   tablespoon Cajun seasoning

1   tablespoon lime juice

1   clove garlic, minced

1   10-ounce package torn European-style salad greens

2   carrots, cut into thin bite-size strips or peeled into thin strips

½ cup thinly sliced radishes

½ cup bottled fat-free ranch salad dressing

Start to Finish: 25 minutes
Makes 4 servings

ONE In a large nonstick skillet cook the French-fried onions over medium-high heat about 2 minutes or until browned, stirring occasionally. Remove from skillet; set aside. **TWO** Trim fat from steak. For rub, in a small bowl combine Cajun seasoning, lime juice, and garlic. Sprinkle evenly over steak; rub in with your fingers. In the same skillet cook steak over medium heat until desired doneness, turning once. (Allow 6 to 8 minutes for medium-rare and 9 to 12 minutes for medium doneness.) Cut steak into thin bite-size slices. If desired, season with salt. **THREE** On a large serving platter toss together the salad greens, carrots, and radishes. Arrange steak strips over greens mixture. Drizzle with dressing. Sprinkle with French-fried onions.

Pork Salad with Cabbage Slaw

Looking for a quick supper on a crisp fall day? Toss pork, apples, and cabbage with a tangy mustard dressing and serve with a loaf of rye bread and mugs of steaming hot cider.

Exchanges: 1 Vegetable, ½ Fruit, 1 Starch, 1½ Lean Meat

Nutrition Facts per serving: 235 cal., 9 g total fat (3 g sat. fat), 56 mg chol., 171 mg sodium, 21 g carbo., 3 g fiber, 19 g pro.
Daily Values: 78% vit. A, 78% vit. C, 5% calcium, 11% iron

1	pound pork loin butterfly chops, cut ¾ inch thick
¼	teaspoon cracked black pepper
⅛	teaspoon ground nutmeg
5	cups packaged shredded cabbage with carrot (coleslaw mix)
1	large apple, coarsely chopped
2	slices turkey bacon or bacon
⅓	cup cider vinegar
⅓	cup apple juice or apple cider
1	tablespoon honey
2	teaspoons honey mustard
1	teaspoon caraway seed

Start to Finish: 30 minutes
Makes 4 servings

ONE Trim fat from chops. Sprinkle chops with pepper and nutmeg. Place chops on the unheated rack of a broiler pan. Broil 3 to 4 inches from the heat for 6 to 8 minutes or until pork is slightly pink in center and juices run clear, turning chops once halfway through broiling. **TWO** Meanwhile, in a large bowl combine cabbage and apple; set aside. In a medium skillet cook bacon over medium heat until crisp. Drain and crumble bacon; set aside. **THREE** In the same skillet combine vinegar, apple juice, honey, honey mustard, and caraway seed. Bring to boiling. Pour over cabbage mixture. Add bacon; toss gently to coat. **FOUR** Divide cabbage mixture among 4 salad plates. Cut pork chops into thin bite-size slices. Arrange pork slices on top of the cabbage mixture.

What Is Cruciferous?

Cabbage, broccoli, Brussels sprouts, cauliflower, and turnips are all members of the family cruciferae. They get their name from the four-petaled flowers that look like a cross. Vegetables from this family might help protect against some forms of cancer because they contain the chemicals beta-carotene and sulforaphane. Sulforaphane also contributes to their distinctive aroma. Cook cruciferous vegetables quickly, uncovered, just until crisp-tender to preserve their mild flavor and to prevent strong-smelling compounds from forming.

Greek Lamb Salad with Yogurt Dressing

Tender lamb, rubbed with fragrant rosemary and garlic, adds Greek inspiration to this invigorating salad. Spinach, cucumber, and golden raisins provide pleasing flavor counterpoints.

Exchanges: 2 Vegetable, 1 Starch, 1½ Lean Meat

Nutrition Facts per serving: 243 cal., 6 g total fat (2 g sat. fat), 36 mg chol., 569 mg sodium, 29 g carbo., 8 g fiber, 20 g pro.
Daily Values: 80% vit. A, 63% vit. C, 17% calcium, 42% iron

8   ounces boneless lamb sirloin chops, cut ¾ inch thick

2   teaspoons snipped fresh rosemary or ½ teaspoon dried rosemary, crushed

1   clove garlic, minced

1   10-ounce package torn fresh spinach or torn mixed salad greens

1   15-ounce can garbanzo beans, rinsed and drained

¼   cup chopped, seeded cucumber

½   cup plain low-fat yogurt

¼   cup chopped green onions

1   clove garlic, minced

⅛   to ¼ teaspoon salt

⅛   teaspoon black pepper

¼   cup golden raisins or dried tart red cherries

Start to Finish: 30 minutes
Makes 4 servings

ONE Trim fat from chops. For rub, in a small bowl combine rosemary and 1 clove garlic. Sprinkle evenly over chops; rub in with your fingers. **TWO** Place chops on the unheated rack of a broiler pan. Broil 3 to 4 inches from the heat for 12 to 15 minutes or until chops are slightly pink in center, turning once halfway through broiling. (Or, grill on the rack of an uncovered grill directly over medium coals for 12 to 14 minutes, turning once halfway through grilling.) Cut chops into thin bite-size slices. **THREE** Meanwhile, in a large bowl toss together the spinach, garbanzo beans, and cucumber. Divide the spinach mixture among 4 salad plates. Arrange lamb slices over spinach mixture. **FOUR** For dressing, in a small bowl combine yogurt, green onions, 1 clove garlic, salt, and pepper. Drizzle dressing over salads. Sprinkle with raisins.

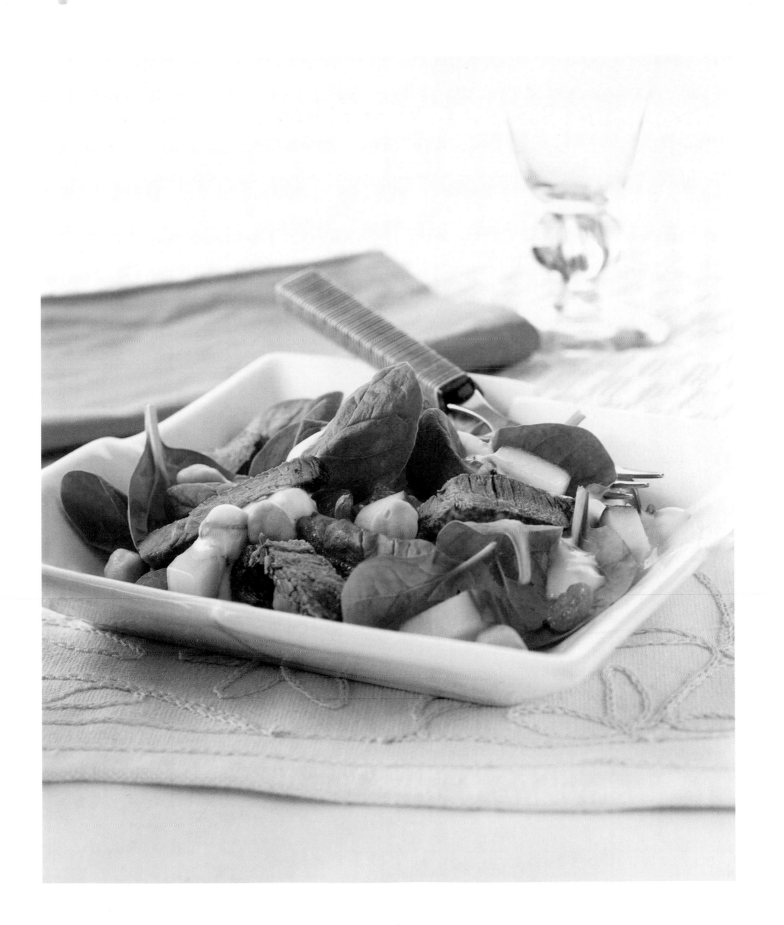

Chicken-Zucchini Salad

When ripe zucchini or summer squash overtake your backyard garden, pick out the best ones to use in this new-style chicken salad. Not a gardener? Drop by your local farmer's market to pick up what you need.

3	cups shredded cooked chicken
1	medium zucchini or yellow summer squash, chopped (1¼ cups)
1	small fennel or kohlrabi bulb, trimmed and chopped (1¼ cups)
4	medium green onions, sliced
1	stalk celery, chopped
1	medium carrot, chopped
2	tablespoons snipped dried apricots (optional)
1	recipe Herbed Mustard Mayonnaise
	Torn salad greens

Prep: 25 minutes
Chill: 4 hours
Makes 6 to 8 servings

ONE In a large bowl combine chicken, zucchini, fennel, green onions, celery, carrot, and, if desired, dried apricots. Pour Herbed Mustard Mayonnaise over chicken mixture; toss gently to coat. Cover and refrigerate for 4 to 24 hours. **TWO** To serve, line 6 to 8 plates with salad greens. Stir chicken mixture; season to taste with salt and black pepper. Spoon the chicken mixture over salad greens.

Herbed Mustard Mayonnaise:
In a small bowl stir together ⅔ cup fat-free or light mayonnaise dressing, 4 teaspoons Dijon-style mustard, 1 tablespoon snipped fresh dill or tarragon, 1 teaspoon finely shredded lemon peel, 1 tablespoon lemon juice, 1 tablespoon frozen orange juice concentrate, and ¼ teaspoon black pepper. Makes about ¾ cup.

Sesame Chicken Salad

Tangy orange juice and mild rice vinegar combine with sesame oil to make an intensely flavored dressing for this unforgettable salad. Toasted sesame oil is available in Asian markets and large grocery stores (see photo, page 51).

Exchanges: 1½ Vegetable, 1 Lean Meat, ½ Fat

Nutrition Facts per serving: 154 cal., 7 g total fat (2 g sat. fat), 53 mg chol., 96 mg sodium, 6 g carbo., 2 g fiber, 15 g pro.
Daily Values: 13% vit. A, 26% vit. C, 3% calcium, 8% iron

1	10-ounce package torn European-style or Italian-style salad greens
2	cups shredded or chopped cooked chicken
1	8¾-ounce can whole baby corn, drained and halved crosswise
2	green onions, sliced
¼	cup sliced radishes
½	cup orange juice
¼	cup rice vinegar or white wine vinegar
½	teaspoon toasted sesame oil
¼	teaspoon black pepper
1½	teaspoons sesame seeds, toasted*

Start to Finish: 20 minutes
Makes 6 servings

ONE In a large bowl combine the salad greens, chicken, baby corn, green onions, and radishes. **TWO** For dressing, in a screw-top jar combine the orange juice, vinegar, sesame oil, and pepper. Cover and shake well. **THREE** Pour dressing over greens mixture; toss gently to coat. Divide among 6 salad bowls. Sprinkle with sesame seeds.

*Note: *To toast sesame seeds, in a nonstick skillet cook and stir sesame seeds over medium heat about 1 minute or just until golden brown. Watch closely so the seeds don't burn. Remove from heat and transfer to a bowl to cool completely.*

Skinny Salad Savvy

Did you know that a build-it-yourself salad from the salad bar can have more calories than a burger, fries, and milk shake? Smart salad builders can take these precautions to keep their salads on the healthful side.

Choose colorful ingredients: *Orange, yellow, and dark green tip you off to vitamin-rich produce.*

Go for the crunch: *Top your salad with chopped fresh veggies, fresh or dried fruit, and nuts or seeds instead of bacon, shredded cheese, fried Chinese noodles, or croutons.*

Drizzle rather than pour: *Choose a reduced-fat dressing and drizzle lightly over your salad, or make your own vinaigrette using 3 parts vinegar to 1 part oil.*

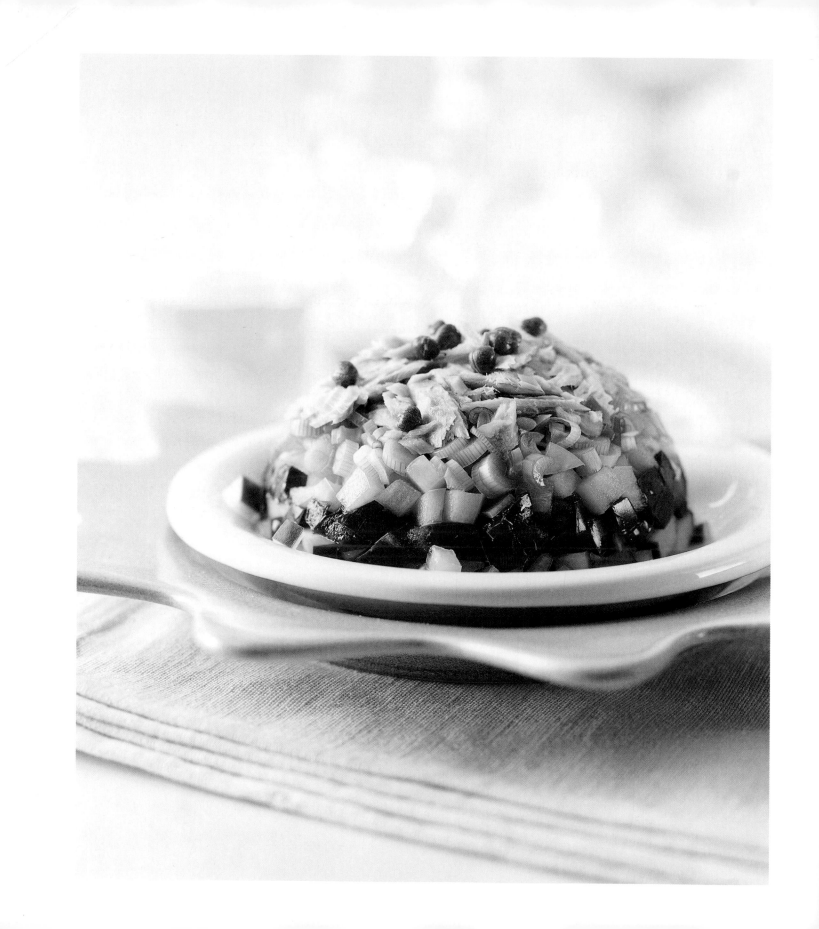

Chopped Salmon Salad

Fresh lemon vinaigrette complements smoky salmon in these stunning but simple layered salads. Serve the chilled entrée with tall glasses of iced tea on a sultry summer evening.

Exchanges: 1 Vegetable, ½ Lean Meat, 1 Fat

Nutrition Facts per serving: 137 cal., 9 g total fat (1 g sat. fat), 8 mg chol., 445 mg sodium, 8 g carbo., 2 g fiber, 8 g pro.
Daily Values: 8% vit. A, 77% vit. C, 1% calcium, 5% iron

¾ cup flaked smoked salmon

¼ cup thinly sliced green onions

½ cup coarsely chopped yellow
sweet pepper

1⅓ cups chopped seeded tomatoes

¼ chopped onion

1 medium cucumber, coarsely
chopped (2 cups)

2 teaspoons small capers, drained

1 recipe Lemon Vinaigrette

Start to Finish: 35 minutes
Makes 4 servings

ONE Line four 6-ounce coffee cups with plastic wrap. Equally divide and layer ingredients in each cup in the following order: salmon, green onions, sweet pepper, tomatoes, onion, and cucumber. Cover with plastic wrap; firmly press mixture into cups with a soup can or similar object slightly smaller than the diameter of the cups. **TWO** To serve, invert cups onto 4 plates; carefully lift off the cups. Remove plastic wrap. Sprinkle with capers. Serve with Lemon Vinaigrette.

Lemon Vinaigrette:
In a screw-top jar combine 2 tablespoons olive oil or salad oil, 2 teaspoons finely shredded lemon peel, 2 tablespoons lemon juice, ½ teaspoon sugar, ¼ teaspoon salt, and several dashes bottled hot pepper sauce. Shake well before serving.

Honey-Glazed Tuna and Greens

The slightly bitter flavor of mesclun contrasts beautifully with the lightly caramelized honey and soy glaze. Swordfish steaks make a tasty substitute for the tuna but are not as rich in omega-3 fatty acids.

Exchanges: 3 Vegetable, 1 Starch, 2 Lean Meat

Nutrition Facts per serving: 279 cal., 2 g total fat (0 g sat. fat), 24 mg chol., 1,015 mg sodium, 22 g carbo., 1 g fiber, 42 g pro.
Daily Values: 9% vit. A, 21% vit. C, 2% calcium, 35% iron

¼ cup honey

¼ cup reduced-sodium soy sauce

1 teaspoon toasted sesame oil

½ teaspoon crushed red pepper

4 5-ounce fresh tuna steaks, cut ½ to 1 inch thick

1 10-ounce package mesclun or torn mixed bitter salad greens

10 to 12 yellow or red tiny pear-shaped tomatoes, halved

Start to Finish: 25 minutes
Makes 4 servings

ONE In a small bowl combine honey, soy sauce, sesame oil, and red pepper. Remove 2 tablespoons to brush on the fish and reserve the remaining mixture for dressing. **TWO** Rinse fish; pat dry with paper towels. Brush both sides of the fish with the 2 tablespoons soy mixture. **THREE** Grill fish on the greased rack of an uncovered grill directly over medium coals until fish flakes easily when tested with a fork (allow 4 to 6 minutes per ½-inch thickness of fish), gently turning 1-inch steaks halfway through grilling. [Or, broil on the greased unheated rack of a broiler pan about 4 inches from the heat (allow 4 to 6 minutes per ½-inch thickness of fish), gently turning 1-inch steaks halfway through broiling.] **FOUR** In a large bowl toss together the mesclun and tomatoes. Divide mesclun mixture among 4 salad plates. Cut fish across the grain into ½-inch slices; arrange over mesclun mixture. Drizzle with the reserved soy mixture.

Asian-Style Shrimp and Millet Salad

Raw millet looks like yellow mustard seeds, but when cooked, it explodes into a fluffy, pale yellow grain that's packed with protein, mincrals, and fiber. Look for millet in health food stores.

Exchanges: ½ Fruit, 1 Starch, 1½ Lean Meat, 1½ Fat

Nutrition Facts per serving: 383 cal., 15 g total fat (2 g sat. fat), 113 mg chol., 226 mg sodium, 43 g carbo., 5 g fiber, 20 g pro.
Daily Values: 40% vit. A, 28% vit. C, 5% calcium, 21% iron

1	tablespoon salad oil
1	cup millet
2	cups water
2	cups peeled and deveined, cooked shrimp
1	medium mango, seeded, peeled, and chopped
1	8-ounce can sliced water chestnuts, drained
¼	cup chopped red onion
¼	cup snipped fresh cilantro
¼	cup rice vinegar
3	tablespoons salad oil
1	tablespoon finely shredded orange peel
1	teaspoon toasted sesame oil
¼	teaspoon salt

Prep: 35 minutes
Chill: 4 hours
Makes 5 or 6 servings

ONE In a large saucepan heat the 1 tablespoon salad oil over medium heat. Add millet; cook and stir for 2 minutes. Carefully add the water. Bring to boiling; reduce heat. Simmer, covered, about 25 minutes or until millet is fluffy and water is absorbed. **TWO** Transfer millet to a large bowl. Add shrimp, mango, water chestnuts, onion, and cilantro; toss gently to combine. **THREE** For dressing, in a small bowl stir together vinegar, the 3 tablespoons salad oil, the orange peel, sesame oil, and salt. Pour over millet mixture; toss gently to coat. Cover and refrigerate for 4 to 24 hours.

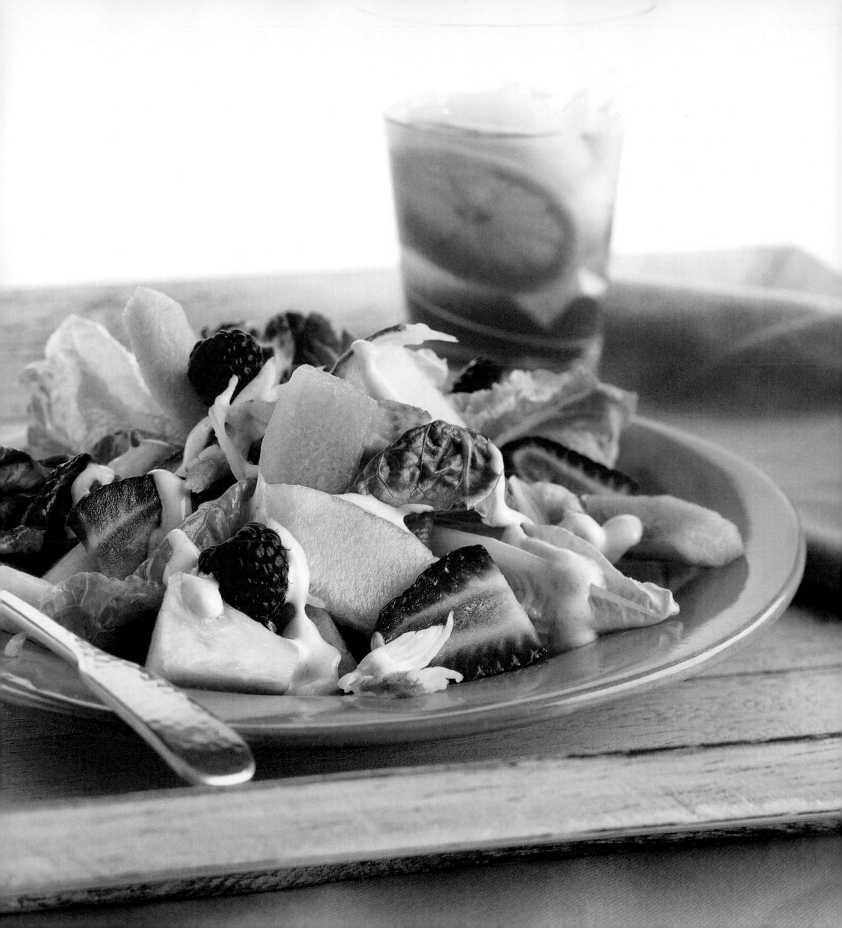

Curried Crab Salad

No doubt about it—this vibrant seafood salad is sure to become a weeknight favorite. You need just 20 minutes to enhance juicy, fresh fruit and crabmeat with a light, curry-seasoned dressing.

Exchanges: 1 Vegetable, 1 Fruit, 1 Lean Meat, 1 Fat

Nutrition Facts per serving: 200 cal., 9 g total fat (2 g sat. fat), 58 mg chol., 361 mg sodium, 17 g carbo., 2 g fiber, 14 g pro.
Daily Values: 21% vit. A, 62% vit. C, 11% calcium, 9% iron

---

2   cups cut-up fresh fruit (such as pineapple, cantaloupe, honeydew melon, and/or strawberries) and/or raspberries

6   ounces cooked crabmeat, cut into bite-size pieces; or one 6-ounce can crabmeat, drained, flaked, and cartilage removed; or one 6-ounce package frozen crabmeat, thawed

³/₄   cup sliced celery

¹/₄   cup light mayonnaise dressing or salad dressing

¹/₄   cup plain low-fat yogurt

2   tablespoons fat-free milk

¹/₂   teaspoon curry powder

4   cups torn mixed salad greens

Start to Finish: 20 minutes
Makes 3 servings

ONE In a large bowl combine fresh fruit, crabmeat, and celery; set aside. **TWO** For dressing, in a small bowl stir together mayonnaise dressing, yogurt, milk, and curry powder. **THREE** Divide greens among 3 salad plates. Top with crab mixture and drizzle with dressing.

Choose Your Crab

Crab, famous for its sweet, succulent meat, is available in a variety of forms—frozen, pasteurized, or canned. Canned crab is available as claw meat, lump meat, or flaked meat. To make this salad as pictured, look for cooked crab legs in your grocery store or seafood shop. About half of the weight of crab legs is shell and cartilage, so purchase twice the required amount of crab meat (12 ounces of cooked crab legs yields 6 ounces of meat). Use a nutcracker to crack each leg joint and remove the meat with a cocktail fork. Use freshly cooked crab within 2 days or freeze the meat for up to 1 month. You may want to use Surimi—an imitation crabmeat made from pollock or another mild-flavored fish. It is lower in cholesterol than crabmeat and costs a fraction of the price.

four.beef, pork, and lamb

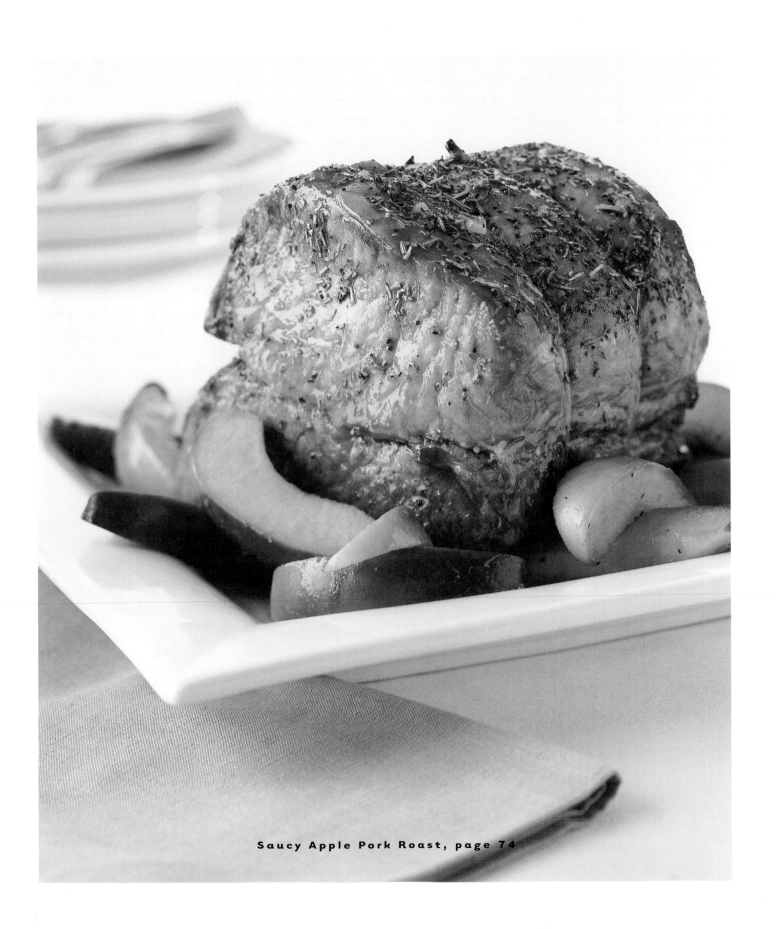

Saucy Apple Pork Roast, page 74

Deviled Roast Beef

Dijon mustard makes this roast a devilish delight. The mustard is rubbed over the meat before roasting and is the star of the flavor-packed mushroom and onion sauce.

Exchanges: 2 Lean Meat

Nutrition Facts per serving: 217 cal., 9 g total fat (3 g sat. fat), 78 mg chol., 342 mg sodium, 5 g carbo., 0 g fiber, 28 g pro.
Daily Values: 4% vit. C, 2% calcium, 22% iron

1	2- to 2½-pound boneless beef eye round roast
¼	cup Dijon-style mustard
¼	teaspoon coarsely ground black pepper
2	cups sliced fresh mushrooms
1	cup beef broth
1	small onion, cut into thin wedges
¼	cup water
2	cloves garlic, minced
1	teaspoon Worcestershire sauce
¼	teaspoon dried thyme, crushed
½	cup fat-free milk
3	tablespoons all-purpose flour

Prep: 20 minutes
Roast: 1½ hours
Stand: 15 minutes
Makes 8 to 10 servings

ONE Trim fat from meat. In a small bowl stir together 2 tablespoons of the mustard and the pepper; spread evenly over meat. Place meat on a rack in a shallow roasting pan. Insert a meat thermometer. **TWO** Roast, uncovered, in a 325° oven until the meat thermometer registers 140° for medium-rare (1½ to 2 hours) or 155° for medium doneness (1¾ to 2¼ hours). Remove meat from oven. Cover meat with foil; let stand for 15 minutes before carving. (The internal temperature will rise about 5° during standing.) **THREE** Meanwhile, for sauce, in a medium saucepan combine the mushrooms, beef broth, onion, water, garlic, Worcestershire sauce, and thyme. Bring to boiling; reduce heat. Simmer, covered, about 5 minutes or until vegetables are tender. In a small bowl stir together the milk and the remaining mustard; gradually stir into flour. Add to mushroom mixture in saucepan. Cook and stir over medium heat until thickened and bubbly. Cook and stir for 1 minute more. **FOUR** To serve, thinly slice meat across the grain. Arrange meat and vegetables on a serving platter. Spoon some of the sauce over meat. Pass the remaining sauce.

Horseradish Flank Steak

A zesty mustard marinade and a creamy horseradish sauce work together to give this steak plenty of zip. To ensure tender pieces of meat, thinly slice flank steak across the grain.

Exchanges: 2 Lean Meat, ½ Fat

Nutrition Facts per serving: 208 cal., 9 g total fat (3 g sat. fat), 53 mg chol., 398 mg sodium, 6 g carbo., 0 g fiber, 24 g pro.
Daily Values: 3% vit. A, 26% vit. C, 3% calcium, 16% iron

1	1-pound beef flank steak
3	tablespoons Dijon-style mustard
3	tablespoons lemon juice
4½	teaspoons reduced-sodium Worcestershire sauce
⅓	cup fat-free dairy sour cream, fat-free mayonnaise dressing or salad dressing
1	green onion, finely chopped
1	to 2 teaspoons prepared horseradish

Prep: 15 minutes
Marinate: 6 hours
Grill: 12 minutes
Makes 4 servings

ONE Trim fat from steak. Using a sharp knife, score steak by making shallow diagonal cuts at 1-inch intervals in a diamond pattern. Repeat on other side. Place the steak in a plastic bag set in a shallow dish. **TWO** For marinade, in a small bowl combine 2 tablespoons of the mustard, the lemon juice, and Worcestershire sauce. Pour over steak; seal bag. Marinate in the refrigerator for 6 to 24 hours, turning bag occasionally. **THREE** For sauce, in a small bowl combine the remaining mustard, the sour cream, green onion, and horseradish. Cover and refrigerate. Remove from refrigerator about 30 minutes before ready to serve. **FOUR** Drain steak, discarding marinade. Grill steak on the rack of an uncovered grill directly over medium coals until desired doneness, turning once halfway through grilling. (Allow 12 to 14 minutes for medium doneness.) [Or, broil on the unheated rack of a broiler pan 3 to 4 inches from the heat, turning once halfway through broiling. (Allow 12 to 14 minutes for medium doneness.)] **FIVE** To serve, thinly slice steak across the grain. Serve with sauce.

Beef Satay with Spicy Peanut Sauce

For this tongue-tingling dish, thread strips of teriyaki-marinated beef on skewers with sweet pepper and green onion, and grill them over medium coals. Serve the kabobs with a spicy hot peanut sauce.

Exchanges: 1½ Lean Meat, 1 Fat

Nutrition Facts per serving: 217 cal., 10 g total fat (3 g sat. fat), 43 mg chol., 567 mg sodium, 10 g carbo., 1 g fiber, 21 g pro.
Daily Values: 13% vit. A, 45% vit. C, 13% iron

1	1- to 1¼-pound beef flank steak
⅓	cup light teriyaki sauce
½	teaspoon bottled hot pepper sauce
1	red or green sweet pepper, cut into ¾-inch chunks
4	green onions, cut into 1-inch pieces
3	tablespoons reduced-fat or regular peanut butter
2	tablespoons light teriyaki sauce
3	tablespoons water

Prep: 25 minutes
Marinate: 30 minutes
Grill: 3 minutes
Makes 5 servings

ONE Trim fat from steak. Cut steak across the grain into ¼-inch slices. For marinade, in a medium bowl combine the ⅓ cup teriyaki sauce and ¼ teaspoon of the hot pepper sauce. Add steak slices; toss to coat. Cover and marinate in the refrigerator for 30 minutes. If using bamboo skewers, soak them in water for 30 minutes to prevent scorching. **TWO** Drain steak, reserving marinade. On bamboo or metal skewers thread steak slices, accordion-style, alternating with sweet pepper chunks and green onion pieces. Brush with the marinade. **THREE** Grill kabobs on the rack of an uncovered grill directly over medium coals for 3 to 4 minutes or until steak is slightly pink in center, turning once halfway through grilling. (Or, broil on the unheated rack of a broiler pan 4 to 5 inches from the heat about 4 minutes, turning once halfway through broiling.) **FOUR** For peanut sauce, in a small saucepan combine peanut butter, the 2 tablespoons teriyaki sauce, the water, and the remaining ¼ teaspoon hot pepper sauce. Cook and stir over medium heat just until smooth and heated through. Serve the kabobs with peanut sauce.

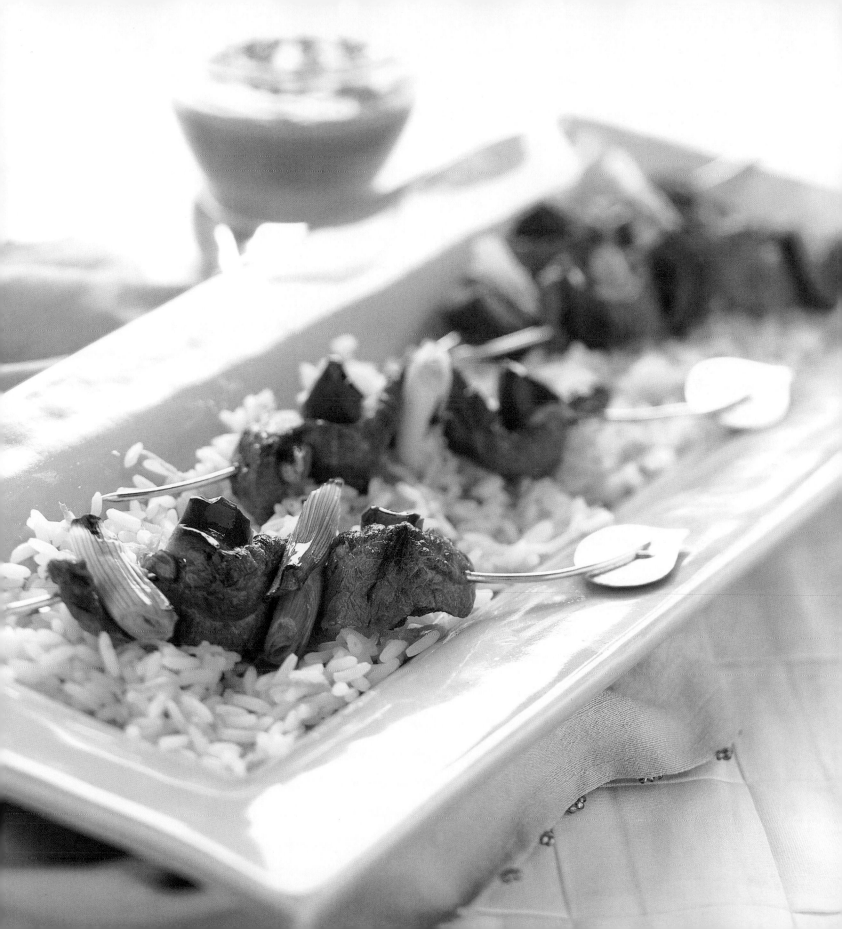

Beef with Mushrooms and Red Wine

The finest flavors of France—Dijon mustard, red wine, and fresh thyme—accent this bistro-style dish. Savor every delectable bite of this seared tenderloin drenched in richly flavored sauce.

Exchanges: 2 Lean Meat, ½ Fat

Nutrition Facts per serving: 263 cal., 14 g total fat (4 g sat. fat), 64 mg chol., 176 mg sodium, 5 g carbo., 1 g fiber, 23 g pro.
Daily Values: 4% vit. C, 1% calcium, 25% iron

4   beef tenderloin steaks, cut ¾ inch thick (about 1 pound total)

1   tablespoon Dijon-style mustard or coarse-grain brown mustard

2   tablespoons olive oil or roasted garlic olive oil

3   cups sliced fresh mushrooms (such as crimini, shiitake, portobello, or button)

⅓   cup dry red wine or dry sherry

1   tablespoon white wine Worcestershire sauce

2   teaspoons snipped fresh thyme

Start to Finish: 20 minutes
Makes 4 servings

ONE Trim fat from steaks. Spread mustard evenly over both sides of steaks. In a large skillet heat 1 tablespoon of the olive oil over medium heat. Add steaks; cook until desired doneness, turning once. (Allow 7 to 10 minutes for medium-rare and 10 to 12 minutes for medium doneness.) Transfer steaks to a serving platter; cover and keep warm.

TWO Add the remaining olive oil to drippings in skillet. Add mushrooms; cook and stir for 4 minutes. Stir in wine, Worcestershire sauce, and thyme. Simmer, uncovered, for 3 minutes more. Spoon the mushroom mixture over steaks.

Beef Goulash Soup

A hint of cocoa lends a new flavor to, and enriches the color of, this favorite Hungarian dish. Cubes of lean sirloin steak cook more quickly than the traditional stew meat does, making this soup suitable for busy weeknights.

Exchanges: 1 Vegetable, ½ Starch, 1 Lean Meat

Nutrition Facts per serving: 178 cal., 6 g total fat (2 g sat. fat), 34 mg chol., 400 mg sodium, 17 g carbo., 2 g fiber, 15 g pro.
Daily Values: 55% vit. A, 47% vit. C, 7% calcium, 18% iron

6	ounces boneless beef sirloin steak
1	teaspoon olive oil
1	medium onion, cut into thin wedges
2	cups water
1	14½-ounce can beef broth
1	14½-ounce can low-sodium tomatoes, undrained and cut up
½	cup thinly sliced carrot
1	teaspoon unsweetened cocoa powder
1	clove garlic, minced
1	cup thinly sliced cabbage
1	ounce dried wide noodles (about ¾ cup)
2	teaspoons paprika
¼	cup fat-free dairy sour cream

Start to Finish: 45 minutes
Makes 4 servings

ONE Trim fat from meat. Cut meat into ½-inch cubes. In a large saucepan heat olive oil over medium-high heat. Add meat. Cook and stir about 3 minutes or until meat is brown. Add onion; cook and stir about 3 minutes more or until onion is tender. **TWO** Stir in the water, beef broth, undrained tomatoes, carrot, cocoa powder, and garlic. Bring to boiling; reduce heat. Simmer, uncovered, about 15 minutes or until the meat is tender. **THREE** Stir in the cabbage, noodles, and paprika. Simmer, uncovered, for 5 to 7 minutes more or until noodles are tender but still firm. Remove from heat. Stir in sour cream.

Beef is Back

Red meat is making a comeback thanks to the popularity of steak houses across the country. Although beef is often listed as a contributer to cardiac-associated health problems, smart choices and right-size portions can help beef fit into a healthy meal plan. Choose from this lean line-up: bottom round roast, top round steak, eye round roast, arm pot roast, round tip roast, top loin steak, and sirloin steak. And remember to keep portion sizes to no more than 3 to 4 ounces of cooked meat.

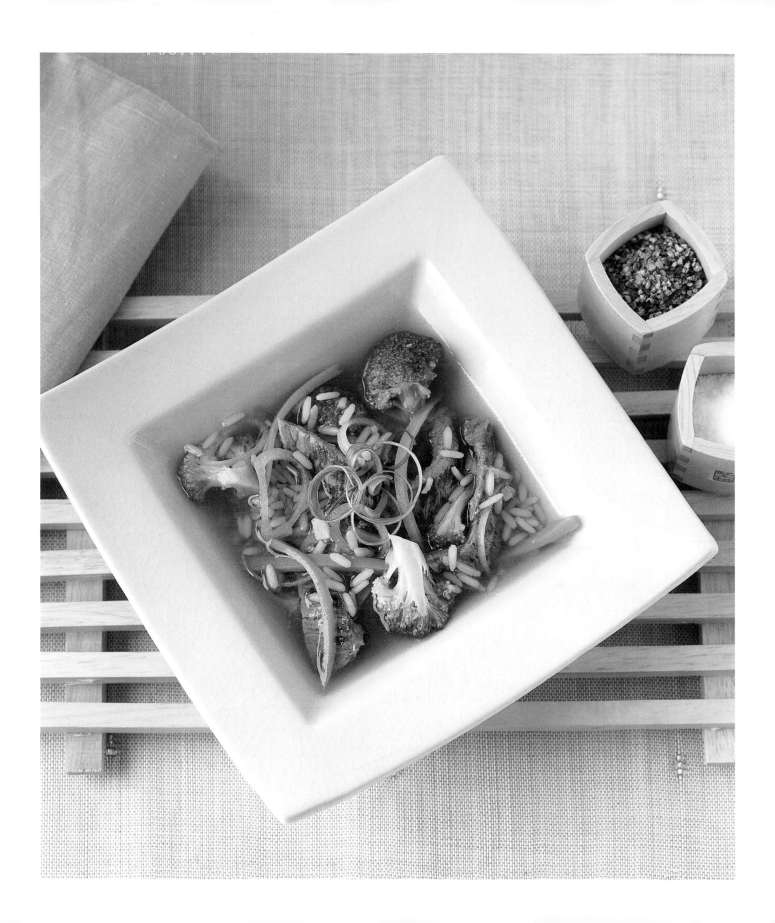

Teriyaki Beef Soup
One serving of this Asian-style soup provides more than half of your daily vitamin C and vitamin A requirements—thanks to the colorful duo of broccoli and carrots.

Exchanges: 2 Vegetable, ½ Starch, 1 Lean Meat

Nutrition Facts per serving: 197 cal., 6 g total fat (2 g sat. fat), 30 mg chol., 382 mg sodium, 22 g carbo., 2 g fiber, 13 g pro.
Daily Values: 76% vit. A, 58% vit. C, 3% calcium, 16% iron

8	ounces boneless beef sirloin steak
2	teaspoons olive oil
1	large shallot, thinly sliced
4	cups water
1	cup apple juice or apple cider
2	carrots, cut into thin bite-size strips
⅓	cup uncooked long grain rice
1	tablespoon grated fresh ginger
3	cloves garlic, minced
1	teaspoon instant beef bouillon granules
2	cups small broccoli flowerets
1	to 2 tablespoons light teriyaki sauce
1	tablespoon dry sherry (optional)
	Slivered green onion tops (optional)

Start to Finish: 40 minutes
Makes 5 servings

ONE Trim fat from meat. Cut meat into thin bite-size strips. In a large saucepan heat olive oil over medium-high heat. Add meat and shallot. Cook and stir for 2 to 3 minutes or until meat is brown. Use a slotted spoon to remove meat mixture; set aside. **TWO** In the same saucepan combine water, apple juice, carrots, rice, ginger, garlic, and bouillon granules. Bring to boiling; reduce heat. Simmer, covered, about 15 minutes or until carrots are tender. **THREE** Stir in the meat mixture and broccoli. Simmer, covered, for 3 minutes more. Stir in the teriyaki sauce and, if desired, the sherry. Ladle soup into bowls. Garnish with slivered green onion tops, if desired.

Saucy Apple Pork Roast

Chunky apple wedges sweetened with brown sugar and apple juice roast alongside an herb-crusted pork loin. For best results, choose firm red apples such as Braeburn or Winesap (see photo, page 65).

Exchanges: ½ Fruit, 2 Lean Meat

Nutrition Facts per serving: 237 cal., 11 g total fat (4 g sat. fat), 72 mg chol., 271 mg sodium, 12 g carbo., 1 g fiber, 23 g pro.
Daily Values: 7% vit. C, 1% calcium, 7% iron

1	3½- to 4-pound boneless pork top loin roast (double loin, tied)
3	cloves garlic, cut into thin slices
1	teaspoon coarse salt or regular salt
1	teaspoon dried rosemary, crushed
½	teaspoon coarsely ground black pepper
3	medium apples, cored and cut into wedges
¼	cup packed brown sugar
¼	cup apple juice or apple cider
2	tablespoons lemon juice
2	teaspoons dry mustard

Prep: 15 minutes
Roast: 1¾ hours
Stand: 10 minutes
Makes 10 to 12 servings

ONE Trim fat from meat. Cut small slits (about ½ inch wide and 1 inch deep) in meat; insert a piece of garlic into each slit. For rub, in a small bowl combine salt, rosemary, and pepper. Sprinkle evenly over meat; rub in with your fingers. Place meat on a rack in a shallow roasting pan. Insert a meat thermometer. Roast, uncovered, in a 325° oven for 1¼ to 1¾ hours or until the meat thermometer registers 145°. Spoon off any fat in roasting pan. **TWO** In a large bowl combine the apples, brown sugar, apple juice, lemon juice, and dry mustard. Spoon the apple mixture around meat. Roast, uncovered, for 30 to 45 minutes more or until meat thermometer registers 155°. **THREE** Transfer meat to a serving platter. Cover meat with foil; let stand for 10 minutes before slicing. (The internal temperature will rise about 5° during standing.) **FOUR** Remove the rack from the roasting pan. Stir the apple wedges into the pan juices. Serve with the meat.

Peachy Pork Tenderloin

You need only five ingredients to prepare this company-special roast. The superb bouquet of peach nectar, rosemary, and grilled pork will entice your guests to the table.

Exchanges: 1½ Lean Meat

Nutrition Facts per serving: 162 cal., 7 g total fat (2 g sat. fat), 60 mg chol., 285 mg sodium, 6 g carbo., 0 g fiber, 19 g pro.
Daily Values: 2% vit. C, 1% calcium, 8% iron

1	12-ounce pork tenderloin
⅓	cup peach nectar
3	tablespoons light teriyaki sauce
2	tablespoons snipped fresh rosemary or 2 teaspoons dried rosemary, crushed
1	tablespoon olive oil

Prep: 10 minutes
Marinate: 4 hours
Grill: 30 minutes
Stand: 10 minutes
Makes 4 servings

ONE Trim fat from meat. Place meat in a plastic bag set in a shallow dish. For marinade, in a small bowl combine peach nectar, teriyaki sauce, rosemary, and olive oil. Pour over meat; seal bag. Marinate in the refrigerator for 4 to 24 hours, turning bag occasionally. Drain meat, discarding the marinade. **TWO** In a grill with a cover arrange medium-hot coals around a drip pan. Test for medium heat above the pan. Place meat on the grill rack directly over drip pan. Cover and grill for 30 to 40 minutes or until meat is slightly pink in center and juices run clear. **THREE** Remove meat from grill. Cover meat with foil; let stand for 10 minutes before slicing.

Fresh Herbs

While other fat-free, sodium-free seasonings might come and go, fresh herbs will always win accolades among health-wise cooks. Packaged fresh herbs are readily available in the produce sections of most supermarkets. To store fresh herbs, place them in a loose-fitting bag in the crisper drawer of your refrigerator. Or trim the stems and place them in a tall container of water, immersing the stems about 2 inches. Cover the leaves loosely with a plastic bag and refrigerate. When you're ready to use the herbs, place a handful of leaves in a measuring cup and snip the herb with kitchen shears.

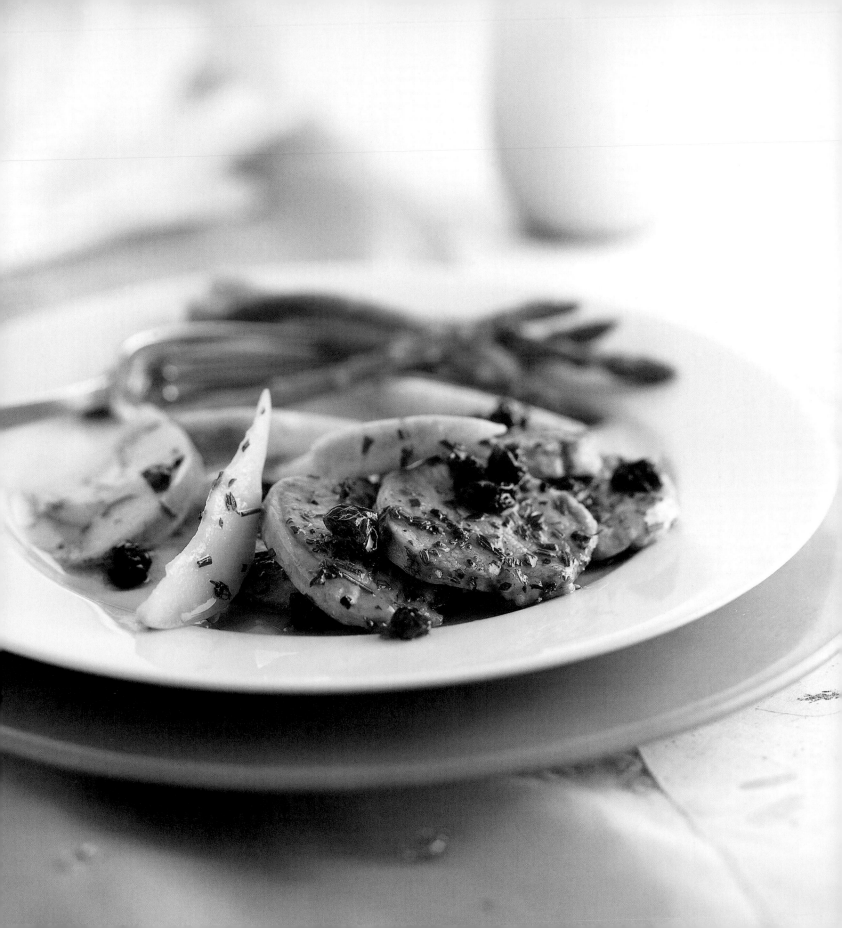

Pork Medallions with Pear Sauce

A fat-free sauce featuring juicy pears, dried tart cherries, maple syrup, and white wine sweetens tender pork medallions scented with rosemary and thyme.

Exchanges: 1½ Fruit, ½ Starch, 1½ Lean Meat

Nutrition Facts per serving: 255 cal., 7 g total fat (2 g sat. fat), 60 mg chol., 179 mg sodium, 29 g carbo., 3 g fiber, 19 g pro.
Daily Values: 2% vit. A, 6% vit. C, 1% calcium, 10% iron

1   12- to 16-ounce pork tenderloin

2   teaspoons snipped fresh rosemary or ½ teaspoon dried rosemary, crushed

1   teaspoon snipped fresh thyme or ¼ teaspoon dried thyme, crushed

¼   teaspoon salt

¼   teaspoon black pepper

1   tablespoon olive oil or cooking oil

2   medium pears, cored and sliced

¼   cup pure maple syrup or maple-flavored syrup

2   tablespoons dried tart red cherries, halved

2   tablespoons dry white wine or apple juice

Start to Finish: 25 minutes
Makes 4 servings

ONE Trim fat from meat. Cut meat into ¼-inch slices. In a medium bowl combine rosemary, thyme, salt, and pepper. Add meat slices; toss to coat. In a large skillet cook meat, half at a time, in hot oil for 2 to 3 minutes or until meat is slightly pink in center, turning once. Remove meat from skillet; set aside. **TWO** In the same skillet combine pears, maple syrup, dried cherries, and white wine. Bring to boiling; reduce heat. Boil gently, uncovered, about 3 minutes or just until pears are tender. Return meat to skillet with pears; heat through. **THREE** To serve, use a slotted spoon to transfer meat to a warm serving platter. Spoon the pear mixture over meat.

Lime Salsa Chops

Marinate boneless pork chops in a fiery mix of hot peppers, lime juice, and cumin to bring the flavors of old Mexico to your dinner table. Lime juice and honey give the salsa a tangy sweetness that's sublime with pork.

Exchanges: 1 Vegetable, 1½ Lean Meat

Nutrition Facts per serving: 211 cal., 18 g total fat (2 g sat. fat), 53 mg chol., 52 mg sodium, 14 g carbo., 1 g fiber, 21 g pro.
Daily Values: 9% vit. A, 25% vit. C, 4% calcium, 7% iron

---

6 boneless pork top loin chops, cut ¾ inch thick

¼ cup finely chopped red onion

¼ cup lime juice

2 fresh serrano or jalapeño peppers, seeded and finely chopped (see tip, page 153)

1 tablespoon toasted sesame oil

1 teaspoon cumin seed, crushed

4 plum tomatoes, chopped

1 small cucumber, seeded and chopped

2 green onions, sliced

2 tablespoons snipped fresh cilantro

1 tablespoon honey

3 tablespoons jalapeño jelly

Prep: 15 minutes
Marinate: 2 hours
Grill: 8 minutes
Makes 6 servings

ONE Trim fat from chops. Place chops in a plastic bag set in a shallow dish. For marinade, in a small bowl combine onion, lime juice, serrano peppers, sesame oil, and cumin seed. Reserve 2 tablespoons of the marinade for salsa. Pour the remaining marinade over chops; seal bag. Marinate in the refrigerator for 2 to 4 hours, turning bag occasionally. **TWO** For salsa, in a medium bowl combine the 2 tablespoons reserved marinade, the tomatoes, cucumber, green onions, cilantro, and honey. Cover and refrigerate until ready to serve. **THREE** Drain chops, reserving marinade. Transfer the marinade to a small saucepan. Add the jalapeño jelly to marinade; cook and stir until mixture boils. Set aside. **FOUR** Grill chops on the rack of an uncovered grill directly over medium coals for 8 to 11 minutes or until chops are slightly pink in center and juices run clear, turning once and brushing occasionally with jelly mixture the last 5 minutes of grilling. (Or, broil on the unheated rack of a broiler pan 3 to 4 inches from the heat for 6 to 8 minutes, turning once and brushing occasionally with jelly mixture the last 5 minutes of broiling.) Serve the chops with salsa.

Chunky Chipotle Pork Chili

Jump-start this aromatic chili with a well-seasoned blend of beer and picante sauce. Add smoky chipotle peppers to round out the flavors. Freeze the remaining chipotle peppers in a freezer container for up to 3 months.

Exchanges: ½ Vegetable, 1 Starch, 1½ Lean Meat

Nutrition Facts per serving: 286 cal., 5 g total fat (1 g sat. fat), 60 mg chol., 778 mg sodium, 31 g carbo., 6 g fiber, 27 g pro.
Daily Values: 16% vit. A, 78% vit. C, 11% calcium, 31% iron

1	12-ounce pork tenderloin
2	teaspoons chili powder
2	teaspoons ground cumin
2	teaspoons cooking oil
1	small onion, chopped
4	cloves garlic, minced
1	yellow or red sweet pepper, cut into ½-inch chunks
1	cup beer or beef broth
½	cup picante sauce or salsa
1	to 2 tablespoons finely chopped canned chipotle peppers in adobo sauce
1	15½-ounce can small red or pinto beans, rinsed and drained
½	cup fat-free or light dairy sour cream
¼	cup snipped fresh cilantro

Start to Finish: 25 minutes
Makes 4 servings

ONE Trim fat from meat. Cut meat into ¾-inch cubes. In a medium bowl combine chili powder and cumin. Add meat cubes; toss to coat. Set aside. **TWO** In a large saucepan heat oil over medium-high heat. Add onion and garlic. Cook and stir about 3 minutes or until onion is tender. Add the meat. Cook and stir about 3 minutes more or until meat is brown. **THREE** Stir in the sweet pepper, beer, picante sauce, and chipotle peppers. Bring to boiling; reduce heat. Simmer, uncovered, about 5 minutes or just until meat is tender. Stir in beans; heat through. **FOUR** To serve, ladle chili into bowls. Top with sour cream and cilantro.

Lamb Chops with Sweet Potato Chutney

Sweet potatoes and dried cranberries make a colorful, richly flavored chutney packed with vitamin A. Serve these petite lamb chops with steamed green beans.

Exchanges: ½ Starch, 2 Lean Meat

Nutrition Facts per serving: 317 cal., 11 g total fat (4 g sat. fat), 97 mg chol., 83 mg sodium, 24 g carbo., 1 g fiber, 30 g pro.
Daily Values: 81% vit. A, 13% vit. C, 3% calcium, 22% iron

8	lamb rib or loin chops, cut 1 inch thick
⅓	cup finely chopped shallots
¼	teaspoon crushed red pepper
¼	cup packed brown sugar
¼	cup vinegar
2	tablespoons dried cranberries or currants
½	teaspoon grated fresh ginger
1	medium sweet potato, peeled and cubed

Start to Finish: 25 minutes
Makes 4 servings

ONE Trim fat from chops. In a small bowl combine the shallots and red pepper. Reserve 2 tablespoons of the shallot mixture for chutney. Sprinkle the remaining shallot mixture evenly over chops; rub in with your fingers. Place chops on the unheated rack of a broiler pan; set aside. **TWO** For chutney, in a medium saucepan combine the 2 tablespoons reserved shallot mixture, the brown sugar, vinegar, cranberries, and ginger. Stir in sweet potato. Bring to boiling; reduce heat. Simmer, covered, for 10 minutes, stirring occasionally. **THREE** Meanwhile, broil chops 3 to 4 inches from the heat until desired doneness, turning chops once halfway through broiling. (Allow 6 to 9 minutes for medium-rare and 7 to 11 minutes for medium doneness.) Serve the lamb chops with the chutney.

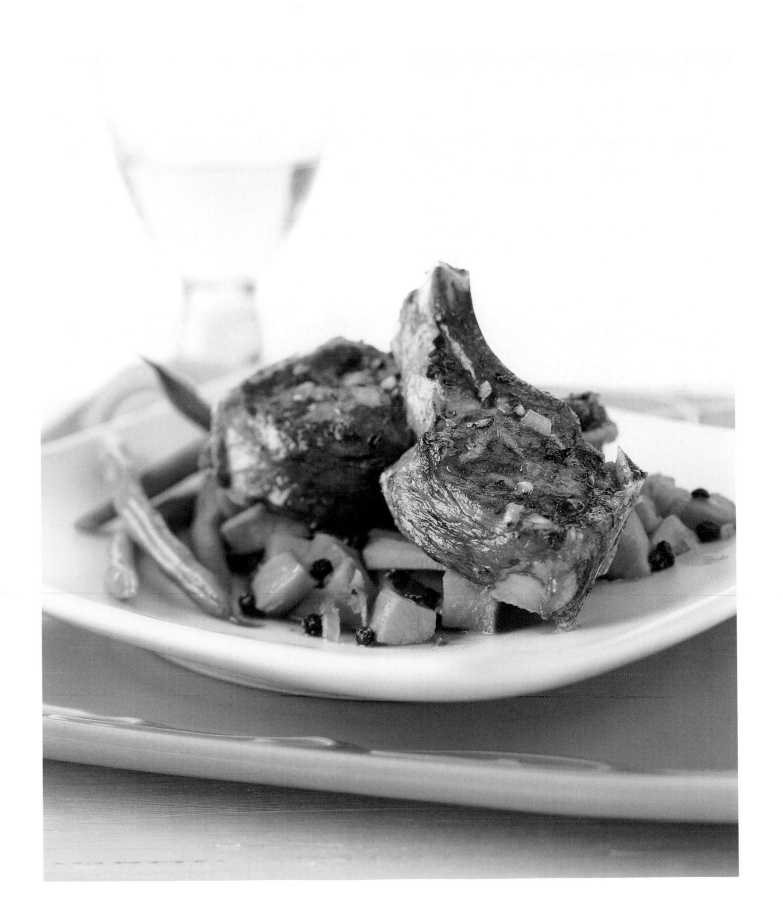

Mint-Rubbed Leg of Lamb

Slivers of garlic tucked into the roast and a rub of mint flavor this springtime classic. Serve the roast medium-rare to medium, in its own juices, with spring vegetables such as asparagus and new potatoes.

Exchanges: 2 Lean Meat

Nutrition Facts per serving: 198 cal., 7 g total fat (2 g sat. fat), 80 mg chol., 169 mg sodium, 6 g carbo., 0 g fiber, 26 g pro.
Daily Values: 5% vit. C, 1% calcium, 17% iron

1	5-pound whole leg of lamb
8	cloves garlic, halved lengthwise
2	tablespoons dried mint, crushed
1	tablespoon coarsely ground black pepper
½	teaspoon salt
3	tablespoons honey

Prep: 20 minutes
Marinate: 2 hours
Roast: 2 hours
Stand: 15 minutes
Makes 10 to 12 servings

ONE Trim fat from meat. Cut 16 small slits (about ½ inch wide and 1 inch deep) in meat; insert a piece of garlic in each slit. **TWO** For rub, in a small bowl combine the mint, pepper, and salt. Sprinkle evenly over meat; rub in with your fingers. Drizzle honey over meat; rub to coat. Place meat on a rack in a shallow roasting pan. Cover meat loosely with plastic wrap; marinate in the refrigerator for 2 hours. **THREE** Remove plastic wrap. Insert a meat thermometer into the thickest part of meat without touching bone. Roast, uncovered, in a 325° oven until the meat thermometer registers 140° for medium-rare (2 to 2½ hours) or 155° for medium doneness (2½ to 3 hours). Remove meat from oven. **FOUR** Cover meat with foil; let stand for 15 minutes before carving. (The internal temperature will rise about 5° during standing.)

Persian-Style Stew

This one-dish crockery cooker dinner of lamb, leeks, split peas, and raisins is perfect for cold winter evenings. During cooking, the yellow split peas soften and thicken the stew to a pleasing consistency.

Exchanges: 1½ Vegetable, 1 Starch, 1½ Lean Meat

Nutrition Facts per serving: 357 cal., 9 g total fat (2 g sat. fat), 58 mg chol., 449 mg sodium, 42 g carbo., 7 g fiber, 29 g pro.
Daily Values: 12% vit. C, 6% calcium, 33% iron

1½	to 2 pounds lamb or beef stew meat
1	tablespoon cooking oil
3	leeks, cut into 1-inch pieces
1	large onion, chopped
½	cup dry yellow split peas
2	bay leaves
4	cloves garlic, sliced
1	tablespoon snipped fresh oregano or 1 teaspoon dried oregano, crushed
1½	teaspoons ground cumin
¼	teaspoon black pepper
3	cups chicken broth
⅓	cup raisins
2	tablespoons lemon juice
3	cups hot cooked bulgur or rice

Prep: 25 minutes
Cook: 4 or 8 hours
Makes 6 to 8 servings

ONE Trim fat from meat. Cut meat into 1-inch cubes. In a large skillet brown meat, half at a time, in hot oil. Drain off fat. **TWO** Transfer meat to a 3½-, 4-, or 5-quart electric crockery cooker. Stir in leeks, onion, split peas, bay leaves, garlic, dried oregano (if using), cumin, and pepper. Pour chicken broth over all. **THREE** Cover and cook on low-heat setting for 8 to 10 hours or on high-heat setting for 4 to 5 hours. **FOUR** If using low-heat setting, turn to high-heat setting. Stir raisins into meat mixture. Cover and cook for 10 minutes more. Discard bay leaves. Stir in lemon juice and, if using, the fresh oregano. To serve, divide the hot bulgur among 6 shallow bowls. Ladle the meat mixture over bulgur.

Keep a Lid on It!

If you are tempted to check the soup or stew in your crockery cooker during the cooking time, resist the urge. An uncovered crockery cooker quickly loses heat, and the lost heat is not readily recovered. An uncovered cooker can lose up to 20° in as little as 2 minutes. So if you lift the cover to add ingredients to your crockery cooker, replace the lid as quickly as possible, especially when cooking on the low-heat setting.

five.poultry

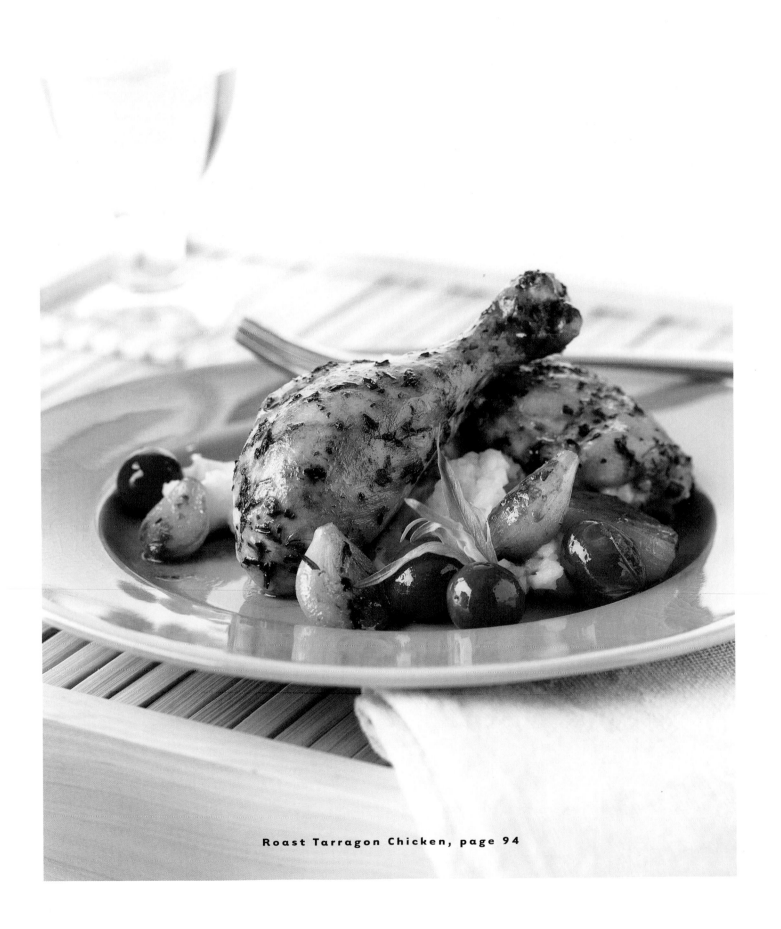

Roast Tarragon Chicken, page 94

Chicken with Pear, Sage, and Cheese

These succulent stuffed chicken breasts can't be beat for simple, healthful, and elegant dining. Juicy pear slices, sharp Romano cheese, and fresh sage are tucked inside the chicken.

Exchanges: 1 Fruit, 2 Lean Meat

Nutrition Facts per serving: 257 cal., 7 g total fat (2 g sat. fat), 82 mg chol., 188 mg sodium, 17 g carbo., 1 g fiber, 29 g pro.
Daily Values: 2% vit. A, 4% vit. C, 8% calcium, 9% iron

---

4   medium skinless, boneless chicken breast halves (about 1 pound total)

1   small Bartlett pear, cored and cut into 8 thin slices

1   ounce Romano or Emmentaler cheese, cut into 4 thin slices

2   tablespoons shredded fresh sage

2   teaspoons olive oil

1½   cups apple juice or apple cider

Start to Finish: 30 minutes
Makes 4 servings

ONE Cut a 3-inch-long pocket into the thick side of each chicken piece. Insert 2 slices of pear and 1 slice of cheese into each pocket. Insert about 1 teaspoon of the sage into each pocket on top of the cheese, reserving the remaining sage. **TWO** In a large skillet cook chicken in hot oil over medium-high heat until brown, turning once. Sprinkle lightly with salt and black pepper. Pour the apple juice over chicken; sprinkle with the reserved sage. Bring to boiling; reduce heat. Simmer, covered, for 7 to 10 minutes or just until chicken is tender and no longer pink. Remove chicken from skillet; cover and keep warm. **THREE** Bring the cooking liquid in skillet to boiling. Boil gently, uncovered, about 5 minutes or until liquid is reduced to about 1 cup. Serve over chicken.

Shredding Herbs

In culinary terms shredded greens or herbs, such as the sage in the recipe above, are referred to as a chiffonade. Chiffonade is a French word translated as "made of rags." To make a chiffonade, stack the herb leaves. Starting at a long edge of the stack, roll the leaves up. With a small, sharp knife, slice the roll into thin strips, about ⅛ inch or thinner. When you're done, you'll have a small pile of herb ribbons. Make a chiffonade of lettuce or other greens in the same manner.

Quick Caribbean Chicken

Sweet potatoes, a frequent ingredient in Caribbean dishes, provide beta-carotene and vitamin C. These two important antioxidants might help protect against disease and slow the aging process.

Exchanges: ½ Fruit, 2 Starch, 1 Lean Meat

Nutrition Facts per serving: 326 cal., 5 g total fat (1 g sat. fat), 45 mg chol., 188 mg sodium, 50 g carbo., 4 g fiber, 20 g pro.
Daily Values: 73% vit. A, 48% vit. C, 3% calcium, 7% iron

12	ounces chicken breast tenderloins or skinless, boneless chicken breast halves, cut lengthwise into 1-inch strips
¼	teaspoon salt
⅛	to ¼ teaspoon ground red pepper
1	teaspoon cooking oil
1	medium sweet potato, peeled, halved lengthwise, and thinly sliced
1	small fresh banana pepper, seeded and chopped
¾	cup unsweetened pineapple juice
1	teaspoon cornstarch
2	unripe bananas, quartered lengthwise and sliced ¾ inch thick
2	cups hot cooked brown rice

Start to Finish: 20 minutes
Makes 4 servings

ONE Sprinkle the chicken strips with salt and red pepper. **TWO** In a large nonstick skillet cook chicken in hot oil over medium heat for 3 minutes. Add the sliced sweet potato and banana pepper. Cook and stir for 5 to 6 minutes more or just until sweet potato is tender. **THREE** Meanwhile, in a small bowl stir together pineapple juice and cornstarch. Add juice mixture to chicken mixture in skillet. Cook until juice mixture is bubbly, stirring gently. Add the banana pieces; cook and stir for 2 minutes more. **FOUR** To serve, divide the hot brown rice among 4 shallow bowls. Top with the chicken mixture.

Summer Chicken and Mushroom Pasta

Healthy doses of garlic and a little white wine perk up this herbed mushroom and pasta combination. Serve this light, fresh dish with a spinach salad and a fruity sorbet for dessert.

Exchanges: 1½ Vegetable, 1 Starch, 1 Lean Meat, ½ Fat

Nutrition Facts per serving: 299 cal., 8 g total fat (2 g sat. fat), 37 mg chol., 249 mg sodium, 33 g carbo., 2 g fiber, 22 g pro.
Daily Values: 5% vit. A, 14% vit. C, 7% calcium, 11% iron

8	ounces dried penne pasta
12	ounces skinless, boneless chicken breast halves, cut into bite-size strips
¼	teaspoon salt
¼	teaspoon freshly ground black pepper
2	tablespoons olive oil or cooking oil
3	large cloves garlic, minced
3	cups sliced fresh mushrooms
1	medium onion, thinly sliced
½	cup chicken broth
¼	cup dry white wine
1	cup cherry tomatoes, halved
¼	cup shredded fresh basil
3	tablespoons snipped fresh oregano
¼	cup shaved Parmesan cheese (optional)

Start to Finish: 30 minutes
Makes 6 servings

ONE Cook pasta in boiling, lightly salted water according to package directions; drain. Return pasta to saucepan; cover and keep warm. **TWO** Meanwhile, sprinkle chicken with salt and ⅛ teaspoon of the pepper. In a large skillet heat 1 tablespoon of the oil over medium-high heat. Add chicken and garlic. Cook and stir for 3 to 4 minutes or until chicken is tender and no longer pink. Remove from skillet; cover and keep warm. **THREE** Add the remaining oil to skillet. Add mushrooms and onion; cook just until tender, stirring occasionally. Carefully add chicken broth and white wine. Bring to boiling; reduce heat. Boil gently, uncovered, about 2 minutes or until liquid is reduced by half. Remove skillet from heat. **FOUR** Add cooked pasta, chicken, cherry tomatoes, basil, and oregano to mushroom mixture; toss gently to coat. Transfer chicken mixture to a serving dish; sprinkle with the remaining ⅛ teaspoon pepper and, if desired, the shaved Parmesan cheese. Serve immediately.

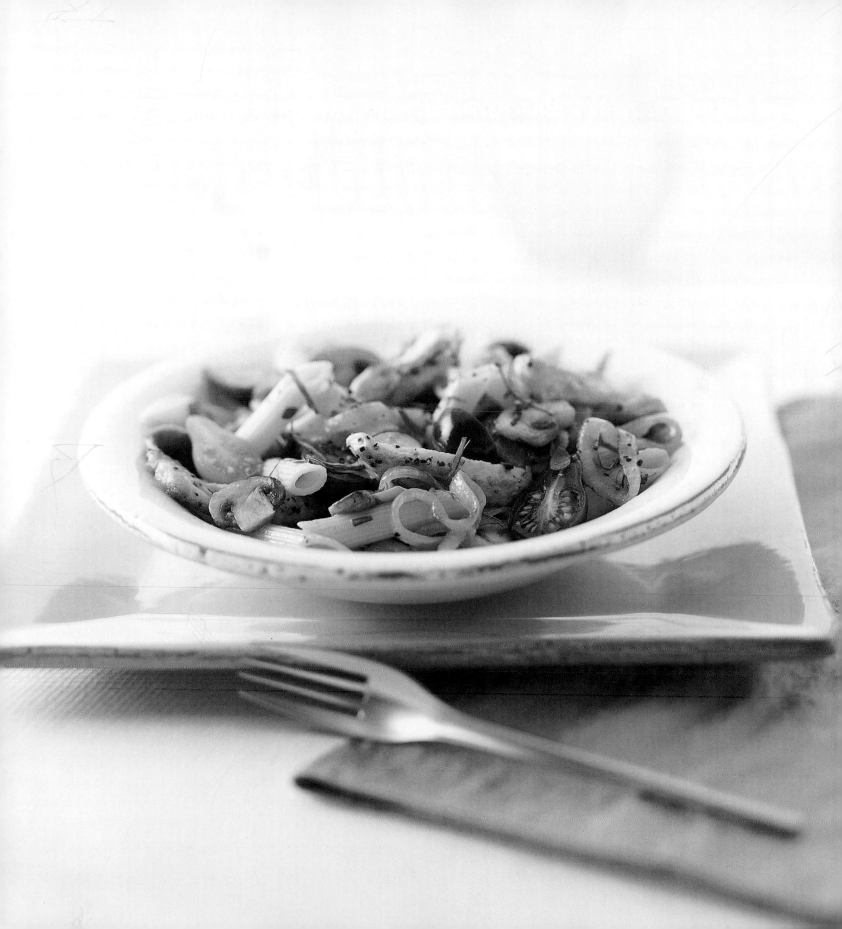

Chicken with Chipotle Barbecue Sauce

Chipotle peppers are dried, smoked jalapeño peppers with a smoky, sweet, almost chocolaty flavor. Here, they lend their distinctive spicy taste to a molasses-sweetened barbecue sauce.

Exchanges: 2 Lean Meat

Nutrition Facts per serving: 291 cal., 6 g total fat (1 g sat. fat), 59 mg chol., 1,399 mg sodium, 36 g carbo., 1 g fiber, 23 g pro.
Daily Values: 101% vit. A, 26% vit. C, 17% iron

¼ cup canned chipotle peppers in adobo sauce

Nonstick cooking spray

⅓ cup finely chopped onion

3 cloves garlic, minced

1 cup catsup

3 tablespoons white wine vinegar

3 tablespoons molasses or sorghum

1 tablespoon Worcestershire sauce

6 medium skinless, boneless chicken breast halves (about 1½ pounds total)

Prep: 30 minutes
Grill: 12 minutes
Makes 6 servings

ONE For sauce, remove any stems from chipotle peppers. Place peppers and adobo sauce in a blender container. Cover and blend until smooth. Set aside. **TWO** Coat a medium saucepan with cooking spray. Heat saucepan over medium heat. Add onion and garlic; cook until onion is tender. Stir in pureed chipotle peppers, catsup, vinegar, molasses, and Worcestershire sauce. Bring to boiling; reduce heat. Simmer, uncovered, about 10 minutes or until the sauce is slightly thickened. **THREE** Grill chicken on the rack of an uncovered grill directly over medium coals for 12 to 15 minutes or until chicken is tender and no longer pink, turning once and brushing occasionally with some of the sauce during the last 5 minutes of grilling. **FOUR** To serve, bring the remaining sauce to boiling. Serve with chicken.

West Indies Chicken with Fruit

Zesty orange marmalade spiked with thyme and coriander glazes these sizzling chicken and fruit kabobs. For best results, choose fruit that is perfectly ripe but firm enough to thread on skewers.

Exchanges: 1½ Fruit, 2 Lean Meat

Nutrition Facts per serving: 288 cal., 7 g total fat (1 g sat. fat), 59 mg chol., 192 mg sodium, 36 g carbo., 3 g fiber, 24 g pro.
Daily Values: 12% vit. A, 142% vit. C, 5% calcium, 11% iron

3	tablespoons orange marmalade
1	tablespoon snipped fresh thyme
2½	teaspoons ground coriander
2	teaspoons finely shredded grapefruit or orange peel
2	teaspoons olive oil
½	teaspoon hot Hungarian paprika or ⅛ teaspoon ground red pepper
¼	teaspoon salt
1	small ruby red grapefruit
2	ripe, yet firm, kiwifruit
2	ripe, yet firm, nectarines
2	ripe, yet firm, carambola (star fruit)
4	medium skinless, boneless chicken breast halves (about 1 pound total)

Prep: 15 minutes
Grill: 12 minutes
Makes 4 servings

ONE For glaze, in a small bowl combine orange marmalade, thyme, coriander, grapefruit peel, oil, paprika, and salt. Set aside. **TWO** Peel and quarter grapefruit and kiwifruit. Pit and quarter nectarines. Cut carambola into ½-inch slices. On 4 metal skewers alternately thread fruits. **THREE** Grill chicken on the rack of an uncovered grill directly over medium coals for 6 minutes. Turn chicken. Place fruit kabobs on grill rack. Brush chicken and fruit with glaze. Grill for 6 to 9 minutes more or until chicken is tender and no longer pink, turning fruit kabobs once and brushing chicken and fruit frequently with glaze.

A Star Is Born

Carambola—a small, oval fruit with deep lengthwise grooves and waxy-looking, bright yellow skin—is a star in the realm of fruit. When ripe, its sweet yellow flesh is juicy and fragrant. Carambola earned its nickname of "star fruit" because when it is cut crosswise, the slices are shaped like stars. Star fruit is available in most grocery stores from late summer to midwinter. Choose fruit that has a bright, even color. Ripen fruit with green tips at room temperature.

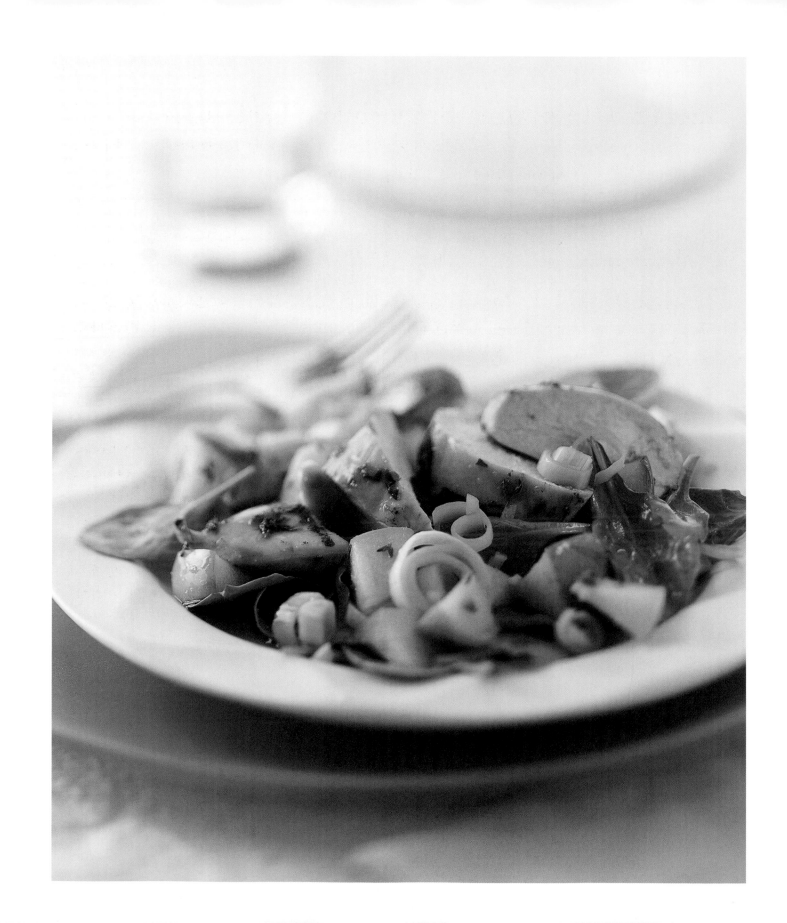

Chicken with Braised Spinach and Leek

A drizzle of lemon-infused apple jelly glazes the broiled chicken and lightly sweetens the spinach. Packaged, prewashed spinach keeps your time in the kitchen to a minimum.

Exchanges: 2 Vegetable, ½ Fruit, 1 Lean Meat

Nutrition Facts per serving: 263 cal., 3 g total fat (1 g sat. fat), 45 mg chol., 654 mg sodium, 42 g carbo., 4 g fiber, 19 g pro.
Daily Values: 48% vit. A, 27% vit. C, 24% iron

½ cup apple jelly

2 tablespoons soy sauce

1 tablespoon snipped fresh thyme
 or 1 teaspoon dried thyme,
 crushed

1 teaspoon grated fresh ginger

1 teaspoon finely shredded lemon
 peel

4 small skinless, boneless chicken
 breast halves (about 12 ounces
 total)

 Nonstick cooking spray

2 medium apples, coarsely chopped

1 medium leek (white part only),
 sliced, or ⅓ cup chopped onion

2 cloves garlic, minced

2 tablespoons apple juice or
 chicken broth

1 10-ounce package torn fresh
 spinach

 Prep: 20 minutes
 Broil: 12 minutes
 Makes 4 servings

ONE For glaze, in a small saucepan heat apple jelly, soy sauce, thyme, ginger, and lemon peel just until jelly is melted. Remove from heat. Remove ¼ cup of the glaze for dressing. **TWO** Place chicken on the unheated rack of a broiler pan. Broil 4 to 5 inches from the heat for 12 to 15 minutes or until chicken is tender and no longer pink, turning and brushing once with the remaining glaze halfway through broiling. (Or, grill on the rack of an uncovered grill directly over medium coals for 12 to 15 minutes, turning and brushing once with the remaining glaze halfway through grilling.) **THREE** Meanwhile, coat a large saucepan or Dutch oven with cooking spray. Heat saucepan over medium heat. Add apples, leek, and garlic; cook for 3 minutes. Add the reserved ¼ cup glaze and the apple juice. Bring to boiling. Add spinach; toss just until wilted. Season to taste with salt and black pepper. **FOUR** To serve, cut each chicken piece crosswise into 6 to 8 slices. Divide the spinach mixture among 4 dinner plates. Top with sliced chicken.

Roast Tarragon Chicken

The bold, aniselike flavor of tarragon complements the sweetness of roasted cherry tomatoes and shallots. If tarragon is too pungent for your taste buds, try rosemary or thyme instead (see photo, page 85).

Exchanges: ½ Vegetable, 1½ Lean Meat, 1 Fat

Nutrition Facts per serving: 227 cal., 13 g total fat (2 g sat. fat), 67 mg chol., 170 mg sodium, 5 g carbo., 1 g fiber, 23 g pro.
Daily Values: 7% vit. A, 26% vit. C, 2% calcium, 8% iron

3 tablespoons olive oil

2½ teaspoons dried tarragon, crushed

2 cloves garlic, minced

½ teaspoon coarsely ground black pepper

¼ teaspoon salt

1 pound cherry tomatoes

8 small shallots

2½ to 3 pounds meaty chicken pieces (breasts, thighs, and drumsticks)

Fresh tarragon (optional)

Prep: 15 minutes
Roast: 45 minutes
Makes 6 servings

ONE In a medium bowl stir together olive oil, tarragon, garlic, pepper, and salt. Add tomatoes and shallots; toss gently to coat. Use a slotted spoon to remove tomatoes and shallots from bowl, reserving the olive oil mixture. **TWO** If desired, skin chicken. Place chicken in a shallow roasting pan. Brush chicken with the reserved olive oil mixture. **THREE** Roast chicken in a 375° oven for 20 minutes. Add the shallots; roast for 15 minutes. Add the tomatoes; roast for 10 to 12 minutes more or until chicken is tender and no longer pink and vegetables are tender. Garnish with fresh tarragon, if desired.

Chicken and Garbanzo Bean Soup

Fresh fennel infuses this hearty soup with its licoricelike flavor. When buying fennel, look for firm, smooth bulbs without cracks or brown spots. Fennel should have crisp stalks and fresh, bright green leaves.

Exchanges: 1 Vegetable, ½ Starch, 1 Lean Meat

Nutrition Facts per serving: 205 cal., 4 g total fat (1 g sat. fat), 40 mg chol., 625 mg sodium, 23 g carbo., 9 g fiber, 20 g pro.
Daily Values: 149% vit. A, 12% vit. C, 6% calcium, 18% iron

1	cup dry garbanzo beans (chickpeas)
1	pound skinless, boneless chicken breast halves or thighs
2½	cups sliced carrots
1	medium fennel bulb, trimmed and cut into ¼-inch slices, or 1½ cups sliced celery
1	large onion, chopped
1	tablespoon snipped fresh marjoram or 1 teaspoon dried marjoram, crushed
1	tablespoon snipped fresh thyme or 1 teaspoon dried thyme, crushed
1	tablespoon instant chicken bouillon granules
¼	teaspoon salt
¼	teaspoon black pepper
4	cups water
1	cup shredded fresh spinach or escarole

Prep: 30 minutes
Soak: 1 hour
Cook: 4 or 8 hours
Makes 6 servings

ONE Rinse garbanzo beans. In a large saucepan combine beans and enough water to cover the beans by 2 inches. Bring to boiling; reduce heat. Simmer, uncovered, for 10 minutes. Remove from heat. Cover and let stand for 1 hour. Drain and rinse beans. **TWO** Place beans and chicken in a 3½-, 4-, or 5-quart electric crockery cooker. Add the carrots, fennel, onion, dried marjoram and thyme (if using), bouillon granules, salt, and pepper. Add the 4 cups water. **THREE** Cover and cook on low-heat setting for 8 to 10 hours or on high-heat setting for 4 to 5 hours. Remove the chicken; cool slightly. Cut the chicken into bite-size pieces. Return to cooker. Stir in the spinach and, if using, the fresh marjoram and thyme. Let stand 5 minutes before serving.

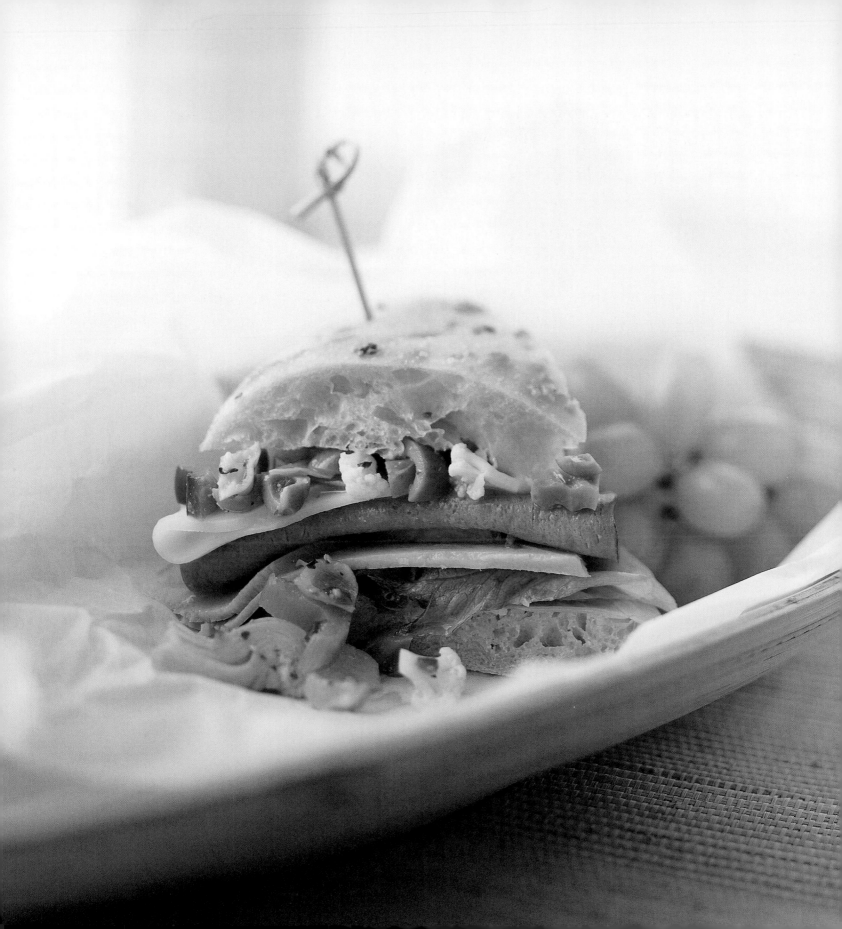

Muffuletta

Fans of this renowned New Orleans sandwich will love this slimmed-down version. Sliced focaccia bursts with smoked lean turkey breast, turkey salami, provolone cheese, artichoke hearts, and piquant giardiniera.

Exchanges: 2 Starch, 1 Lean Meat, ½ Fat

Nutrition Facts per serving: 275 cal., 9 g total fat (3 g sat. fat), 45 mg chol., 1,262 mg sodium, 27 g carbo., 1 g fiber, 21 g pro.
Daily Values: 2% vit. A, 2% vit. C, 25% calcium, 8% iron

1	12-inch Italian flat bread (focaccia)
	Lettuce leaves
6	ounces thinly sliced mesquite-smoked turkey breast
4	ounces thinly sliced reduced-fat salami or sliced cooked turkey salami
5	ounces thinly sliced reduced-fat provolone or mozzarella cheese
⅓	cup giardiniera (pickled mixed vegetables) or pepperoncini salad peppers, drained and chopped
¼	cup chopped pitted green olives
¼	cup thinly sliced canned artichoke hearts
¼	cup bottled fat-free Italian salad dressing

Prep: 20 minutes
Makes 6 servings

ONE Cut focaccia in half horizontally. Layer ingredients on bottom half of focaccia in the following order: lettuce, turkey, salami, and cheese. **TWO** In a small bowl combine giardiniera, olives, artichoke hearts, and salad dressing; spoon evenly over cheese. Add the top half of focaccia. Wrap securely in plastic wrap and refrigerate up to for 4 hours before serving.

Cool, Clear Water

Our bodies are at least 60 percent fluid. That's why we need 8 to 12 eight-ounce glasses of fluids daily. Johns Hopkins Weight Management Center recommends individuals drink at least eight glasses of water daily before drinking other beverages (such as coffee or soda). Water is a natural appetite suppressant and an important part of healthier eating. Make it easy to get enough water by keeping a filled water bottle or glass always within reach.

Wild Rice Chicken Soup

A splash of Madeira enhances chicken and rice soup with rich yet mellow flavor. If you have leftover roast chicken, use 1½ cups chopped cooked chicken in place of the frozen chicken breast.

Exchanges: 1 Vegetable, 2 Starch, ½ Lean Meat

Nutrition Facts per serving: 236 cal., 5 g total fat (1 g sat. fat), 38 mg chol., 440 mg sodium, 31 g carbo., 2 g fiber, 18 g pro.
Daily Values: 10% vit. A, 48% vit. C, 2% calcium, 16% iron

1	6.2-ounce package quick-cooking long grain and wild rice mix
2	14½-ounce cans reduced-sodium chicken broth
1	tablespoon snipped fresh thyme or 1 teaspoon dried thyme, crushed
4	cloves garlic, minced
4	cups chopped tomatoes
1	9-ounce package frozen chopped cooked chicken breast
1	cup finely chopped zucchini
¼	teaspoon freshly ground black pepper
1	tablespoon Madeira or dry sherry (optional)

Start to Finish: 25 minutes
Makes 6 servings

ONE Prepare rice mix according to package directions, except omit the seasoning packet and the margarine. **TWO** Meanwhile, in a Dutch oven combine the chicken broth, dried thyme (if using), and garlic. Bring to boiling. Stir in the tomatoes, chicken, zucchini, pepper, and if using, fresh thyme. **THREE** Return to boiling; reduce heat. Simmer, covered, for 5 minutes. Stir in cooked rice and, if desired, Madeira. Heat through.

Asian-Style Turkey

Embellish these orange- and ginger-marinated turkey kabobs with a spoonful of Fruit Salsa in a Big Way (see recipe, page 153) and serve the colorful skewers on a bed of brown rice.

Exchanges: 1½ Lean Meat

Nutrition Facts per serving: 132 cal., 3 g total fat (1 g sat. fat), 50 mg chol., 389 mg sodium, 1 g carbo., 0 g fiber, 22 g pro.
Daily Values: 4% vit. C, 1% calcium, 7% iron

---

1   pound turkey breast tenderloin steaks or skinless, boneless chicken breast halves

¼   cup dry white wine

¼   cup orange juice

¼   cup soy sauce

2   tablespoons water

1   tablespoon rice vinegar

1   tablespoon cooking oil

1   teaspoon garlic powder

1   teaspoon ground ginger

Prep: 20 minutes
Marinate: 4 hours
Broil: 8 minutes
Makes 4 servings

ONE Cut turkey lengthwise into thin strips. Place turkey in a plastic bag set in a shallow dish. **TWO** For marinade, in a 2-cup glass measure combine white wine, orange juice, soy sauce, water, rice vinegar, oil, garlic powder, and ginger. Pour over turkey; seal bag. Marinate in the refrigerator for 4 hours, turning bag occasionally. If using bamboo skewers, soak them in water for 30 minutes to prevent scorching. **THREE** Drain turkey, discarding marinade. On bamboo or metal skewers thread turkey strips, accordion-style. **FOUR** Place kabobs on the unheated rack of a broiler pan. Broil 4 to 5 inches from the heat for 8 to 10 minutes or until turkey is tender and no longer pink, turning once halfway through broiling.

Alcohol Alternatives

Adding alcohol to recipes is a favorite way to enhance flavors, especially in low-fat dishes. Although the alcohol content of one serving of most foods is a fraction of that found in a typical beverage containing alcohol, those wishing to avoid all alcohol can easily make substitutions. For dry white wine, use chicken or vegetable broth, ginger ale, white grape juice, or diluted apple cider vinegar. For dry red wine, try beef, chicken, or vegetable broth; tomato juice; grape or cranberry juice with a dash of lemon; or diluted red wine vinegar. For beer, acceptable substitutions are chicken broth, white grape juice, or ginger ale.

Turkey Mushroom Marsala

If you like, spoon the golden brown turkey and the herbed mushroom sauce over hot cooked linguine. Tally ¾ cup cooked pasta as 105 calories or 1½ starch exchanges.

Exchanges: 1½ Lean Meat

Nutrition Facts per serving: 151 cal., 5 g total fat (1 g sat. fat), 50 mg chol., 114 mg sodium, 1 g carbo., 0 g fiber, 22 g pro.
Daily Values: 1% vit. C, 1% calcium, 10% iron

4	4-ounce turkey breast tenderloin steaks
1	cup sliced fresh shiitake mushrooms
⅓	cup dry Marsala
⅓	cup water
1½	teaspoons snipped fresh thyme or ½ teaspoon dried thyme, crushed
1	teaspoon snipped fresh rosemary or ¼ teaspoon dried rosemary, crushed
⅛	teaspoon salt
⅛	teaspoon black pepper
2	teaspoons olive oil or cooking oil
2	teaspoons cold water
1	teaspoon cornstarch
	Hot cooked linguine (optional)
	Fresh thyme (optional)

Prep: 15 minutes
Marinate: 30 minutes
Cook: 15 minutes
Makes 4 servings

ONE Place turkey in a plastic bag set in a shallow dish. For marinade, in a small bowl combine the mushrooms, Marsala, the ⅓ cup water, the thyme, rosemary, salt, and pepper. Pour over turkey; seal bag. Marinate in the refrigerator for 30 minutes to 2 hours, turning bag occasionally. **TWO** Drain turkey, reserving marinade. Pat turkey dry with paper towels. In a large skillet heat oil over medium heat. Add turkey. Cook for 8 to 10 minutes or until turkey is tender and no longer pink, turning once. Remove turkey from skillet; cover and keep warm. **THREE** Pour the marinade into skillet. Bring to boiling; reduce heat. Simmer, covered, for 2 minutes. **FOUR** Stir together the 2 teaspoons cold water and the cornstarch; stir into marinade in skillet. Cook and stir over medium heat until thickened and bubbly. Cook and stir for 2 minutes more. If desired, serve the turkey and mushroom mixture over linguine and garnish with fresh thyme.

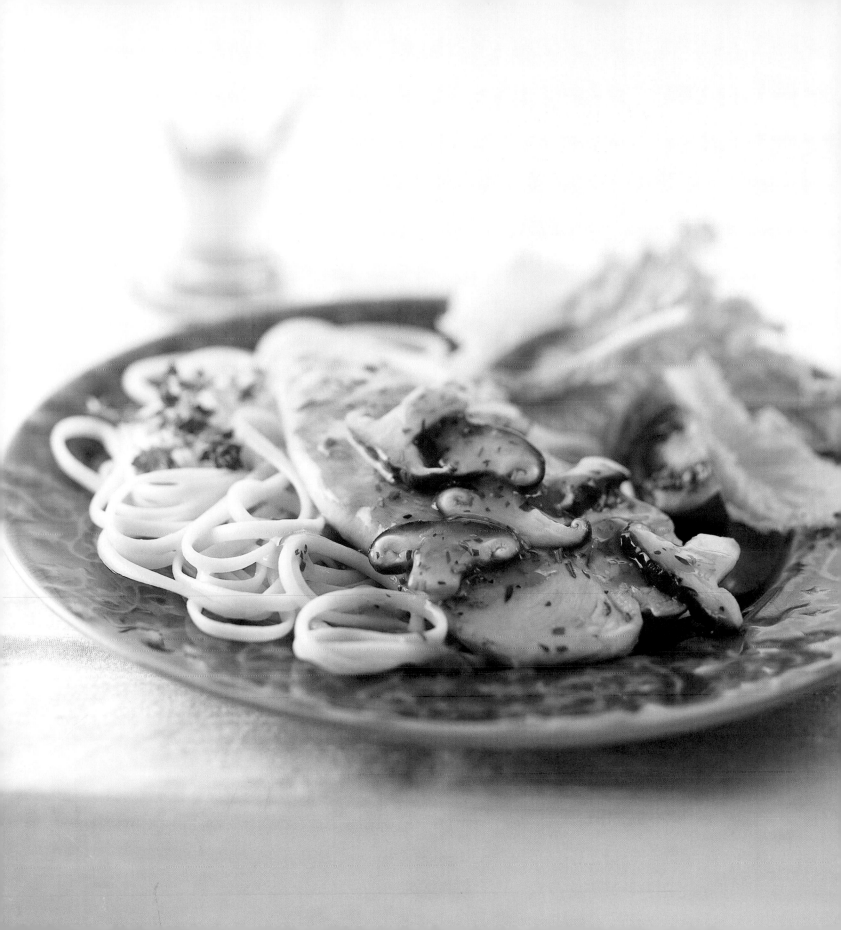

Turkey Piccata with Fettuccine
Ready in 30 minutes, this elegant dish allows you to dine in style any night of the week. The delicate wine sauce made from the pan drippings is heavenly when served with the pan-fried turkey steaks.

Exchanges: 1 Starch, 1½ Lean Meat, 1 Fat

Nutrition Facts per serving: 331 cal., 10 g total fat (2 g sat. fat), 50 mg chol., 292 mg sodium, 31 g carbo., 0 g fiber, 26 g pro.
Daily Values: 1% vit. A, 21% vit. C, 2% calcium, 18% iron

4 ounces dried fettuccine or linguine

¼ cup all-purpose flour

½ teaspoon lemon-pepper seasoning or black pepper

4 4-ounce turkey breast tenderloin steaks

2 tablespoons olive oil or cooking oil

⅓ cup dry white wine

2 tablespoons lemon juice

2 tablespoons water

½ teaspoon instant chicken bouillon granules

1 tablespoon capers, rinsed and drained (optional)

2 tablespoons snipped fresh parsley

Start to Finish: 30 minutes
Makes 4 servings

ONE Cook pasta according to package directions; drain. Return to saucepan; cover and keep warm. **TWO** Meanwhile, in a small bowl stir together flour and lemon-pepper seasoning. Place each turkey steak between 2 pieces of plastic wrap. Using the flat side of a meat mallet, pound to ⅛-inch thickness. Dip the turkey steaks into the flour mixture to coat. **THREE** In a 12-inch skillet heat oil over medium-high heat. Add turkey. Cook about 4 minutes or until turkey is tender and no longer pink, turning once. Remove turkey from skillet; cover and keep warm. **FOUR** For sauce, add the wine, lemon juice, water, and bouillon granules to skillet, scraping up crusty bits from bottom of pan. If desired, stir in capers. Bring to boiling; reduce heat. Simmer, uncovered, for 2 minutes. Remove from heat; stir in snipped parsley. **FIVE** To serve, divide the pasta among 4 dinner plates. Top with the turkey and the sauce.

Turkey and Soba Noodle Stir-Fry

With a beguiling and nutty flavor, Japanese soba noodles (also called buckwheat noodles) are increasingly popular. They contain more protein and fiber than most noodles.

Exchanges: ½ Vegetable, 2 Starch, 1 Lean Meat

Nutrition Facts per serving: 331 cal., 6 g total fat (1 g sat. fat), 37 mg chol., 384 mg sodium, 48 g carbo., 3 g fiber, 25 g pro.
Daily Values: 18% vit. A, 110% vit. C, 4% calcium, 22% iron

6	ounces dried soba (buckwheat) noodles or whole wheat spaghetti
2	teaspoons cooking oil
2	cups sugar snap peas
1	medium red sweet pepper, cut into thin strips
4	green onions, bias-sliced into 1-inch pieces
12	ounces turkey breast tenderloin steaks, cut into bite-size strips
1	teaspoon toasted sesame oil
½	cup bottled plum sauce
¼	teaspoon crushed red pepper

Start to Finish: 25 minutes
Makes 4 servings

ONE Cook soba noodles according to package directions; drain. Return to saucepan; cover and keep warm. **TWO** Meanwhile, pour cooking oil into a wok or large skillet. (Add more oil as necessary during cooking.) Preheat over medium-high heat. Stir-fry snap peas and sweet pepper in hot oil for 2 minutes. Add green onions. Stir-fry for 1 to 2 minutes more or until vegetables are crisp-tender. Remove vegetables from wok. **THREE** Add turkey and sesame oil to the hot wok. Stir-fry for 3 to 4 minutes or until turkey is tender and no longer pink. Add plum sauce and crushed red pepper. Return cooked vegetables to wok; stir to coat ingredients with sauce. Heat through. Serve immediately over soba noodles.

six.fish and seafood

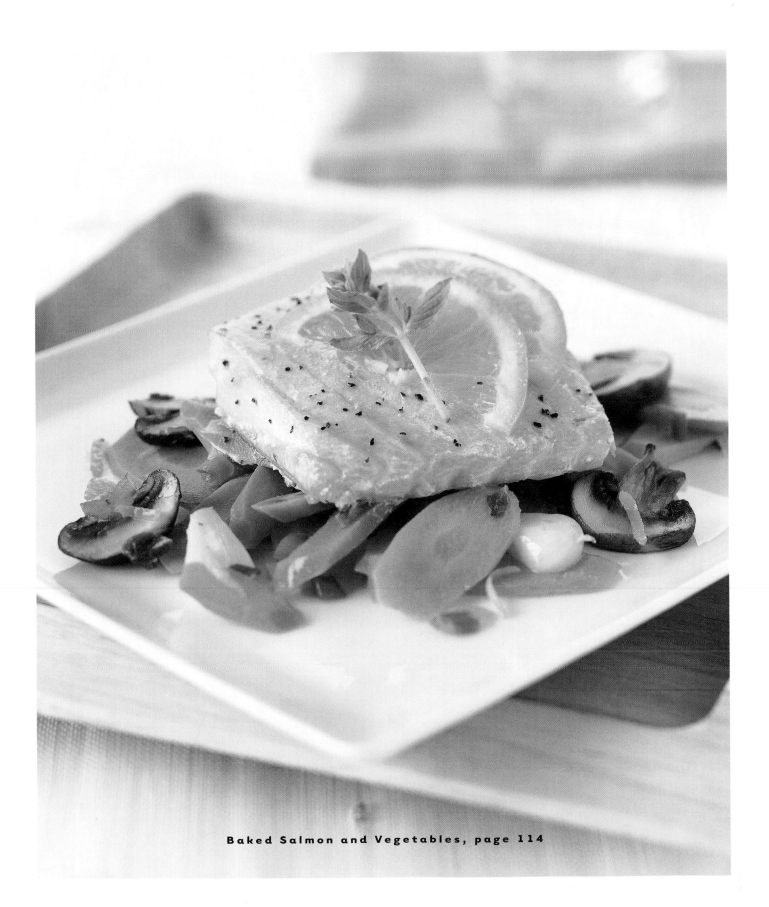

Baked Salmon and Vegetables, page 114

Orange Roughy with Nectarine Salsa

Make orange roughy the light, healthful star of your next barbecue. Let the lean, delicate fish shine with a topping of salsa made from refreshing cucumbers and ripe, juicy nectarines.

Exchanges: ½ Fruit, 1½ Lean Meat

Nutrition Facts per serving: 158 cal., 3 g total fat (1 g sat. fat), 60 mg chol., 97 mg sodium, 10 g carbo., 1 g fiber, 22 g pro.
Daily Values: 6% vit. A, 55% vit. C, 3% calcium, 5% iron

1	1-pound fresh or frozen orange roughy fillet, 1 inch thick
1	large nectarine, cut into ½-inch pieces
1	small cucumber, seeded and cut into ½-inch pieces
1	kiwifruit, peeled and cut into ½-inch pieces
¼	cup thinly sliced green onions
3	tablespoons orange juice
1	tablespoon white wine vinegar
1	teaspoon olive oil
½	teaspoon freshly ground black pepper

Prep: 15 minutes
Grill: 8 minutes
Makes 4 servings

ONE Thaw fish, if frozen. **TWO** For salsa, in a medium bowl combine nectarine, cucumber, kiwifruit, green onions, orange juice, and vinegar. Cover and refrigerate until ready to serve. **THREE** Rinse fish; pat dry with paper towels. Drizzle fish with oil; rub in with your fingers. Sprinkle with pepper. **FOUR** Place fish in a well-greased wire grill basket. Grill fish on the rack of an uncovered grill directly over medium coals for 8 to 12 minutes or until fish flakes easily when tested with a fork, turning basket once halfway through grilling. **FIVE** To serve, cut fish into 4 serving-size pieces. Spoon the salsa over fish.

Citrus-Honey Swordfish

You'll find many uses for this versatile five-ingredient marinade. Its sweet, tangy flavor also complements grilled or broiled chicken, pork, and other firm fleshed fish.

Exchanges: 1 Starch, 2 Lean Meat

Nutrition Facts per serving: 303 cal., 6 g total fat (1 g sat. fat), 34 mg chol., 550 mg sodium, 34 g carbo., 1 g fiber, 27 g pro.
Daily Values: 3% vit. A, 20% vit. C, 1% calcium, 14% iron

1	pound fresh or frozen swordfish steaks, cut 1 inch thick
¼	cup orange juice
2	tablespoons lemon juice
2	tablespoons Dijon-style mustard
2	tablespoons honey
1	tablespoon soy sauce
4	ounces dried vermicelli

Prep: 15 minutes
Marinate: 1 hour
Grill: 8 minutes
Makes 4 servings

ONE Thaw fish, if frozen. Rinse fish; pat dry with paper towels. Cut fish into 4 serving-size pieces. Place fish in a plastic bag set in a shallow dish. **TWO** For marinade, in a small bowl combine orange juice, lemon juice, mustard, honey, and soy sauce. Pour over fish; seal bag. Marinate in the refrigerator for 1 to 2 hours, turning bag occasionally. Drain fish, reserving marinade. **THREE** Grill fish on the greased rack of an uncovered grill directly over medium coals for 8 to 12 minutes or until fish flakes easily when tested with a fork, gently turning and brushing once with some of the marinade halfway through grilling. Transfer the remaining marinade to a small saucepan. Bring to boiling. **FOUR** Meanwhile, cook pasta according to package directions; drain. Toss the pasta with heated marinade. Serve with fish.

The Fish Switch

Can't find red snapper at your grocery store? A finicky eater won't eat tuna? Make the fish switch. Choose a comparable substitute from the list below. Make sure you purchase a similar thickness and trade a fillet for a fillet—not a fillet for a steak—so the cooking time in the recipe will work for your new selection.

Instead of:	Try:
orange roughy	cod, flounder, sea bass, sole
red snapper	trout, whitefish
swordfish	tuna, sea bass, shark
salmon	swordfish, tuna
tuna	mackerel, salmon, swordfish

Tuna with Fresh Orange Salsa

A robustly flavored cumin rub on the tuna pairs wonderfully with the vibrant orange and tomato salsa. Toasted walnuts lend a surprise crunch to the salsa.

Exchanges: 1 Fruit, 1½ Lean Meat

Nutrition Facts per serving: 262 cal., 12 g total fat (2 g sat. fat), 43 mg chol., 343 mg sodium, 11 g carbo., 3 g fiber, 28 g pro.
Daily Values: 74% vit. A, 76% vit. C, 5% calcium, 10% iron

4	fresh or frozen tuna or sea bass steaks, cut 1 inch thick
1	teaspoon finely shredded orange peel
4	medium oranges, peeled, sectioned, and coarsely chopped
1	large tomato, seeded and chopped
¼	cup snipped fresh cilantro
2	tablespoons thinly sliced green onion
2	tablespoons chopped walnuts, toasted (see tip, page 152)
1	tablespoon lime juice
½	teaspoon ground cumin
½	teaspoon salt
½	teaspoon black pepper
1	tablespoon olive oil

Prep: 20 minutes
Broil: 8 minutes
Makes 4 servings

ONE Thaw fish, if frozen. **TWO** For the orange salsa, in a medium bowl combine the orange peel, chopped oranges, tomato, cilantro, green onion, walnuts, lime juice, ¼ teaspoon of the salt, and ¼ teaspoon the pepper. Set aside. **THREE** Rinse fish; pat dry with paper towels. In a small bowl combine cumin, the remaining ¼ teaspoon salt, and the remaining ¼ teaspoon pepper. Brush the fish with olive oil and sprinkle evenly with cumin mixture. **FOUR** Place fish in a well-greased wire grill basket. Grill fish on the rack of an uncovered grill directly over medium coals for 8 to 12 minutes or until fish flakes easily when tested with a fork, turning basket once halfway through grilling. (Or, place fish on the greased unheated rack of a broiler pan. Broil about 4 inches from the heat for 8 to 12 minutes or until fish flakes easily when tested with a fork, gently turning once halfway through broiling.) Spoon the orange salsa over fish.

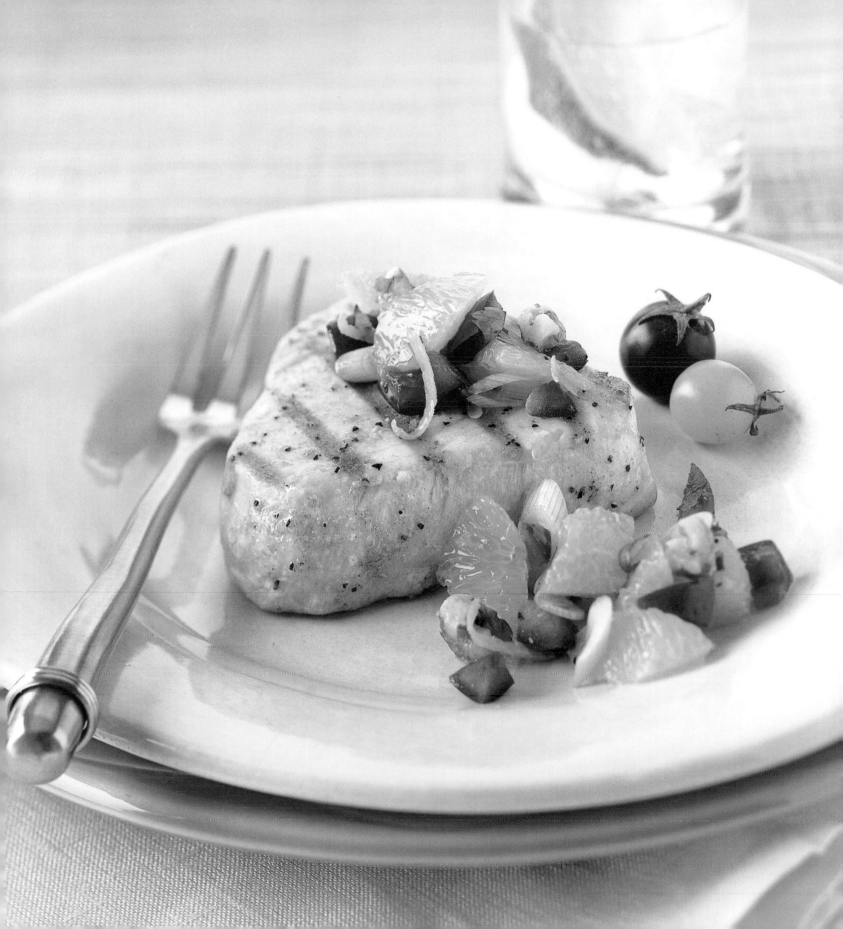

Mango-Sauced Red Snapper

Wake up your palate with the contrast of fiery-hot crushed red pepper and sweet summer fruit. If fresh mangoes are not available, look for a jar of refrigerated mango slices in the produce section of your grocery store.

Exchanges: ½ Fruit, 2½ Lean Meat

Nutrition Facts per serving: 322 cal., 11 g total fat (2 g sat. fat), 18 mg chol., 309 mg sodium, 18 g carbo., 2 g fiber, 37 g pro.
Daily Values: 36% vit. A, 25% vit. C, 5% calcium, 3% iron

4	6-ounce fresh or frozen skinless red snapper fillets, ½ inch thick
¼	teaspoon crushed red pepper
1	tablespoon margarine or butter
½	cup finely chopped onion
1½	teaspoons cornstarch
¼	teaspoon crushed red pepper
⅔	cup chicken broth
1	cup peeled and chopped mango
¼	cup dried tart cherries, snipped
2	tablespoons margarine or butter
	Lime wedges

Start to Finish: 25 minutes
Makes 4 servings

ONE Thaw fish, if frozen. Rinse fish; pat dry with paper towels. Sprinkle the fish with ¼ teaspoon crushed red pepper; set aside. **TWO** For sauce, in a small saucepan melt the 1 tablespoon margarine over medium heat. Add the onion; cook until tender. Stir in the cornstarch and ¼ teaspoon crushed red pepper. Add chicken broth all at once. Cook and stir until thickened and bubbly. Add mango and dried cherries; cook and stir for 2 minutes more. Remove from heat. Cover and keep warm. **THREE** In a 12-inch nonstick skillet melt the 2 tablespoons margarine over medium-high heat. Add the fish. Cook for 4 to 6 minutes or until fish flakes easily when tested with a fork, gently turning once. **FOUR** To serve, arrange the fish on a serving platter. Spoon the sauce over fish. Serve with lime wedges.

Managing a Mango

Because the meat from mangoes holds tightly to the seeds, these fruits require persuasion before yielding their fragrant, spicy, peachlike flesh. An easy way to remove the meat is to make a cut through the mango, sliding a sharp knife next to the seed along one side. Repeat on the other side of the seed, resulting in two large pieces. Cut away all of the meat that remains around the oval seed. Remove the peel on all the pieces; cut the fruit as directed.

Smoked Pepper Halibut

Toasted oregano enhances the smoky flavor of spicy chipotle peppers. Toast oregano by stirring it in a dry skillet over medium heat about 1 minute or until it becomes fragrant. Mexican oregano is available in Mexican markets.

Exchanges: ½ Vegetable, 1½ Lean Meat

Nutrition Facts per serving: 133 cal., 3 g total fat (0 g sat. fat), 36 mg chol., 188 mg sodium, 2 g carbo., 1 g fiber, 24 g pro.
Daily Values: 19% vit. A, 41% vit. C, 6% calcium, 6% iron

6	4-ounce fresh or frozen halibut, swordfish, or shark steaks, cut 1 inch thick
1	medium red sweet pepper, cut up
2	canned chipotle peppers in adobo sauce
2	tablespoons adobo sauce
2	tablespoons lime juice
2	cloves garlic, halved
1	teaspoon dried Mexican oregano or regular oregano, toasted
¼	teaspoon salt

Prep: 15 minutes
Marinate: 30 minutes
Grill: 8 minutes
Makes 6 servings

ONE Thaw fish, if frozen. Rinse fish; pat dry with paper towels. Set aside. **TWO** For marinade, in a blender container combine the sweet pepper, chipotle peppers, adobo sauce, lime juice, garlic, and oregano. Cover and blend until pureed. **THREE** Transfer half of the marinade to a shallow glass dish; reserve the remaining marinade until ready to serve. Add the fish steaks to marinade in glass dish, spooning some of the marinade over fish. Cover and marinate at room temperature for 30 minutes. **FOUR** Drain fish, discarding marinade. Sprinkle the fish with salt. Grill fish on the greased rack of an uncovered grill directly over medium coals for 8 to 12 minutes or until fish flakes easily when tested with a fork, gently turning once halfway through grilling. **FIVE** To serve, heat the reserved marinade. Serve with the fish.

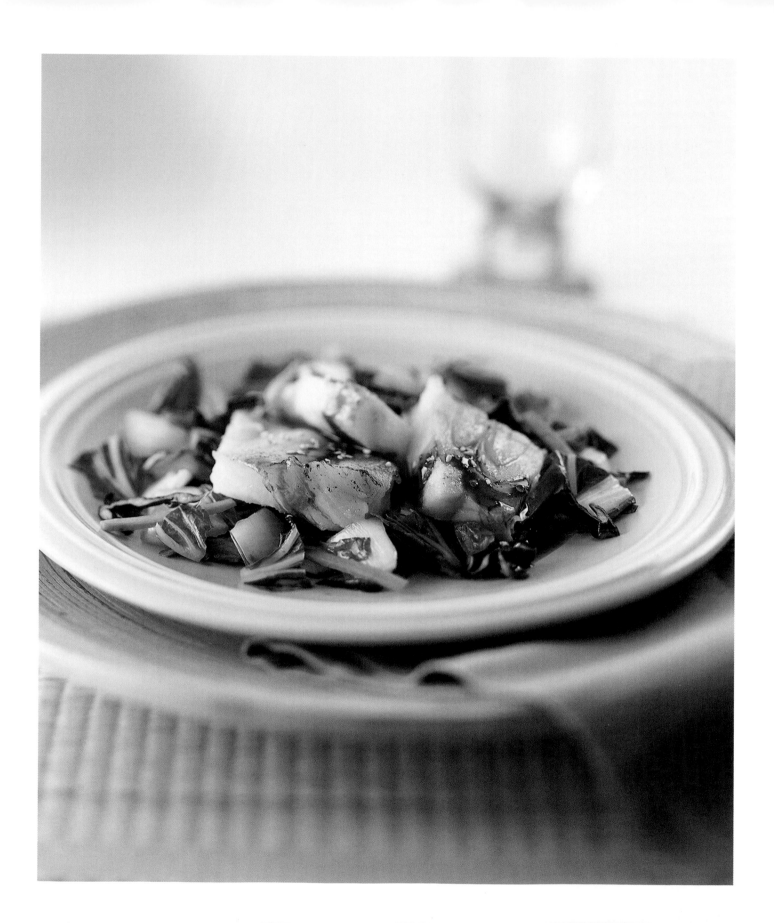

Sesame-Teriyaki Sea Bass

A golden teriyaki glaze and toasted sesame seed transform sea bass fillets into a tantalizing main dish. Serve the fillets on a bed of braised red cabbage, chopped bok choy, and carrot strips as shown in the photo, opposite.

Exchanges: 1½ Lean Meat

Nutrition Facts per serving: 185 cal., 6 g total fat (1 g sat. fat), 47 mg chol., 851 mg sodium, 6 g carbo., 0 g fiber, 22 g pro.
Daily Values: 5% vit. A, 4% vit. C, 1% calcium, 5% iron

4	4-ounce fresh or frozen sea bass fillets, 1 inch thick
¼	teaspoon black pepper
3	tablespoons soy sauce
3	tablespoons sweet rice wine (mirin)
2	tablespoons dry white wine
2½	teaspoons sugar
2½	teaspoons honey
2	teaspoons cooking oil
2	tablespoon white or black sesame seeds, toasted*

Prep: 20 minutes
Cook: 8 minutes
Makes 4 servings

ONE Thaw fish, if frozen. Rinse fish; pat dry with paper towels. Sprinkle the fish with pepper; set aside. **TWO** For glaze, in a small saucepan combine soy sauce, rice wine, dry white wine, sugar, and honey. Bring to boiling; reduce heat. Simmer, uncovered, about 10 minutes or until the glaze is reduced to about ¼ cup. **THREE** Meanwhile, in a large nonstick skillet heat the oil over medium heat. Add the fish. Cook for 8 to 12 minutes or until fish flakes easily when tested with a fork, gently turning once. **FOUR** To serve, arrange the fish on a serving platter. Drizzle the glaze over fish. Sprinkle with sesame seeds.

*Note: To toast sesame seeds, in a nonstick skillet cook and stir sesame seeds over medium heat about 1 minute or just until golden brown. Watch closely so the seeds don't burn. Remove from heat and transfer to a bowl to cool completely.

Baked Salmon and Vegetables

Reminiscent of foil packs from summer camp, this salmon dish is a nearly effortless midweek meal. Oregano and orange slices update the packets with a fresh, new taste (see photo, page 105).

Exchanges: 1 Vegetable, ½ Fruit, 1½ Lean Meat

Nutrition Facts per serving: 226 cal., 9 g total fat (1 g sat. fat), 20 mg chol., 288 mg sodium, 19 g carbo., 5 g fiber, 19 g pro.
Daily Values: 198% vit. A, 71% vit. C, 6% calcium, 14% iron

4	4-ounce fresh or frozen skinless salmon fillets, ¾ inch thick
2	cups thinly bias-sliced carrots
2	cups sliced fresh mushrooms
4	green onions, sliced
2	teaspoons finely shredded orange peel
2	teaspoons snipped fresh oregano or ½ teaspoon dried oregano, crushed
4	cloves garlic, halved
¼	teaspoon salt
¼	teaspoon black pepper
4	teaspoons olive oil
2	medium oranges, thinly sliced
4	sprigs fresh oregano (optional)

Prep: 25 minutes
Bake: 30 minutes
Makes 4 servings

ONE Thaw fish, if frozen. Rinse fish; pat dry with paper towels. Set aside. In a covered small saucepan cook carrots in a small amount of boiling water for 2 minutes. Drain and set aside. Tear off four 24-inch pieces of heavy foil. Fold each piece in half to make an 18×12-inch rectangle. **TWO** In a large bowl combine the carrots, mushrooms, green onions, orange peel, snipped or dried oregano, garlic, salt, and pepper. Divide the vegetable mixture among the foil rectangles. **THREE** Place the fish on top of vegetable mixture. Drizzle the fish with oil; sprinkle lightly with additional salt and black pepper. For each packet, bring up 2 opposite edges of foil and seal with a double fold. Fold remaining ends to completely enclose the food, allowing space for steam to build. Place the foil packets in a single layer in a large baking pan. **FOUR** Bake in a 350° oven about 30 minutes or until fish flakes easily when tested with a fork and carrots are tender. Open packets slowly to allow steam to escape. Transfer the contents of each packet to a dinner plate. Top with orange slices and, if desired, fresh oregano sprigs.

Salmon Steaks with Mustard-Jalapeño Glaze

Wait until the last few minutes of grilling to brush the salmon with the spicy, sweet glaze. Add lengthwise slices of zucchini and sweet pepper halves to the grill for a tasty accompaniment.

Exchanges: 1½ Lean Meat

Nutrition Facts per serving: 213 cal., 7 g total fat (1 g sat. fat), 74 mg chol., 462 mg sodium, 7 g carbo., 1 g fiber, 29 g pro.
Daily Values: 4% vit. A, 20% vit. C, 4% calcium, 10% iron

4   fresh or frozen salmon steaks, cut ¾ inch thick

3   tablespoons Dijon-style mustard

3   canned jalapeño peppers, seeded (if desired) and finely chopped

1   tablespoon frozen orange juice concentrate, thawed

1   tablespoon light-colored corn syrup

½   teaspoon lemon-pepper seasoning

1   teaspoon olive oil

Prep: 15 minutes
Grill: 6 minutes
Makes 4 servings

ONE Thaw fish, if frozen. Rinse fish; pat dry with paper towels. Set aside. **TWO** For glaze, in a small bowl stir together the mustard, jalapeño peppers, orange juice concentrate, corn syrup, and lemon-pepper seasoning. **THREE** Lightly brush both sides of fish with oil. Grill fish on the rack of an uncovered grill directly over medium coals for 6 to 9 minutes or until fish flakes easily when tested with a fork, gently turning once and brushing frequently with glaze during the last 2 to 3 minutes of grilling.

Nothing Fishy Here

Amazing—a fat that is good for you! The omega-3 fatty acids found in cold-water, higher fat varieties of fish, such as sardines, tuna, mackerel, herring, trout, and salmon, are beneficial for reducing the risk of cancer, reducing the symptoms of arthritis, boosting the immune system, reducing high blood pressure, and decreasing the risk of heart disease. Plan on including these smart fish choices in your lineup of meals at least twice each week.

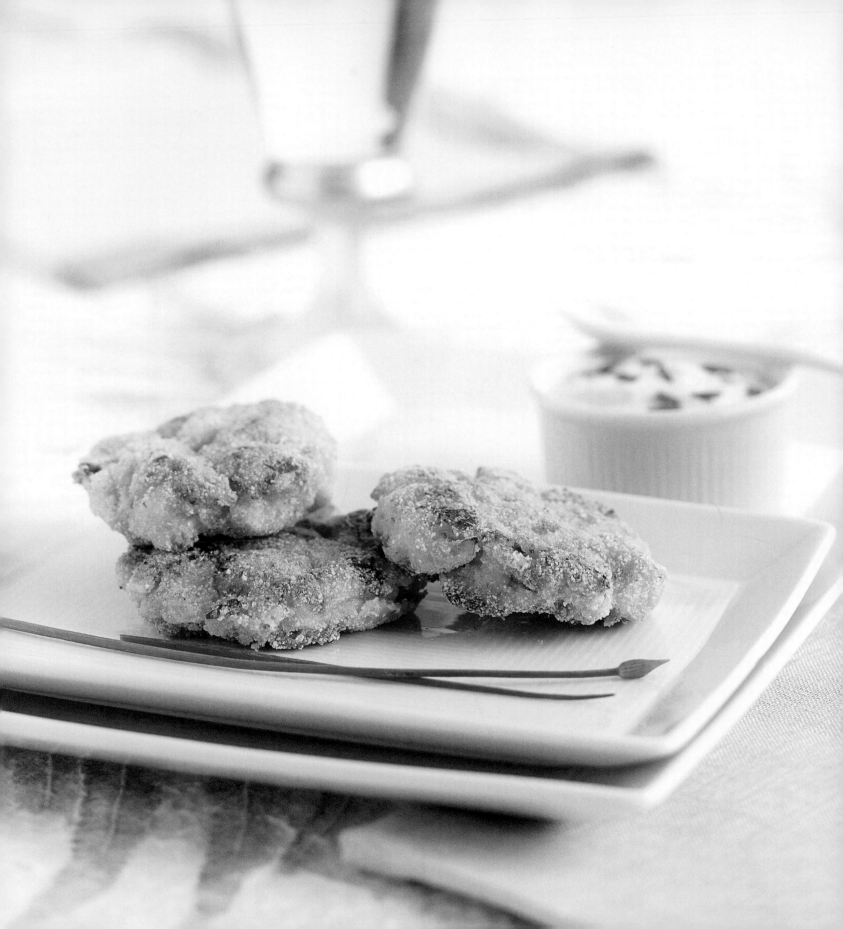

Fish Cakes with Green Goddess Sauce

Hints of tangy lime peel and sharp mustard permeate these cornmeal-coated fish cakes. To keep the meal light, serve it with steamed baby carrots.

Exchanges: 1 Starch, 1 Lean Meat, 1 Fat

Nutrition Facts per serving: 217 cal., 9 g total fat (2 g sat. fat), 109 mg chol., 337 mg sodium, 12 g carbo., 1 g fiber, 20 g pro.
Daily Values: 7% vit. A, 7% vit. C, 9% calcium, 10% iron

12	ounces fresh or frozen skinless white fish fillets (such as haddock or cod)
1	beaten egg
1/4	cup fine dry bread crumbs
2	tablespoons finely chopped onion
4	teaspoons light mayonnaise dressing or salad dressing
1	tablespoon Dijon-style mustard
1	tablespoon snipped fresh parsley
1	teaspoon finely shredded lime peel
1/4	teaspoon salt
2	tablespoons cornmeal
1	tablespoon cooking oil
1	recipe Green Goddess Sauce
	Chives (optional)

Prep: 30 minutes
Cook: 8 minutes
Makes 4 servings

ONE Thaw fish, if frozen. Rinse fish; pat dry with paper towels. Cut fish into 1/2-inch pieces. Set aside. **TWO** In a medium bowl combine egg, bread crumbs, onion, mayonnaise dressing, mustard, parsley, lime peel, and salt. Add fish; mix well. Shape into twelve 1/2-inch-thick patties. Coat both sides of the fish patties with cornmeal. **THREE** In a large nonstick skillet or on a nonstick griddle heat oil over medium heat. Add half of the fish cakes. Cook for 4 to 6 minutes or until fish flakes easily when tested with a fork, gently turning once. Remove from skillet. Repeat with the remaining cakes. Serve with Green Goddess Sauce. If desired, garnish with fresh chives.

Green Goddess Sauce:

In a blender container or food processor bowl combine 1/4 cup plain fat-free yogurt, 1/4 cup light dairy sour cream, and 3 tablespoons snipped fresh tarragon. Cover and blend or process until smooth. Transfer to a small bowl. Stir in 1/4 cup light dairy sour cream, 2 tablespoons snipped fresh chives, 2 teaspoons lime juice, and 1 clove garlic, minced. Store any remaining sauce, covered, in the refrigerator up to 3 days and serve with salad greens. Makes about 3/4 cup.

Thai-Spiced Scallops

These spicy scallop kabobs prove that healthy foods can be packed with great taste. Sea scallops, not to be confused with bay scallops, are the larger of the two varieties.

1	pound fresh or frozen sea scallops
⅔	cup bottled sweet and sour sauce
2	tablespoons snipped fresh basil
1	teaspoon Thai seasoning or five-spice powder
½	teaspoon bottled minced garlic
2	medium yellow summer squash and/or zucchini, quartered lengthwise and sliced ½ inch thick
1½	cups packaged peeled baby carrots

Prep: 20 minutes
Grill: 15 minutes
Makes 4 servings

ONE Thaw scallops, if frozen. Rinse scallops; pat dry with paper towels. Halve any large scallops. On four 8- to 10-inch metal skewers thread scallops. Cover and refrigerate until ready to grill. **TWO** For sauce, in a small bowl combine the sweet and sour sauce, basil, Thai seasoning, and garlic. Remove ¼ cup of the sauce for basting; reserve the remaining sauce until ready to serve. **THREE** Fold a 36×18-inch piece of heavy foil in half to make an 18-inch square. Place squash and carrots in center of foil. Sprinkle lightly with salt and black pepper. Bring up 2 opposite edges of foil and seal with a double fold. Fold remaining ends to completely enclose vegetables, leaving space for steam to build. **FOUR** Grill vegetable packet on the rack of an uncovered grill directly over medium coals for 10 minutes, turning occasionally. **FIVE** Place scallop kabobs on grill rack. Grill for 5 to 8 minutes more or until scallops are opaque and vegetables are crisp-tender, turning kabobs and vegetable packet once and brushing scallops occasionally with the ¼ cup sauce during the last 2 to 3 minutes of grilling. Serve the scallops and vegetables with the remaining sauce.

Grilled Peanut Shrimp Skewers
A quick roast over a fiery grill, and these wondrous kabobs transport you to the Far East with their spicy mix of ginger, cardamom, coriander, cumin, turmeric, and crushed red pepper.

Exchanges: 1½ Lean Meat, ½ Fat

Nutrition Facts per serving: 248 cal., 10 g total fat (2 g sat. fat), 129 mg chol., 180 mg sodium, 22 g carbo., 2 g fiber, 20 g pro.
Daily Values: 5% vit. A, 9% vit. C, 6% calcium, 13% iron

---

1   pound fresh or frozen large shrimp in shells

⅓   cup orange marmalade

2   tablespoons lime juice

2   tablespoons peanut butter

1   tablespoon cooking oil

1   teaspoon grated fresh ginger

1   clove garlic, minced

½   teaspoon ground cardamom

½   teaspoon ground coriander

½   teaspoon ground cumin

¼   teaspoon ground turmeric

⅛   teaspoon ground red pepper

2   tablespoons coconut, toasted

Hot cooked rice (optional)

Prep: 20 minutes
Marinate: 30 minutes
Grill: 10 minutes
Makes 4 servings

ONE Thaw shrimp, if frozen. Peel and devein shrimp. Rinse shrimp; pat dry with paper towels. **TWO** For marinade, in a medium bowl use a wire whisk to combine orange marmalade, lime juice, peanut butter, oil, ginger, garlic, cardamom, coriander, cumin, turmeric, and ground red pepper. Reserve ¼ cup of the marinade until ready to serve. Add shrimp to the remaining marinade; toss to coat. Cover and marinate at room temperature for 30 minutes, stirring occasionally. **THREE** Drain shrimp, discarding marinade. On 4 long metal skewers thread shrimp. Grill shrimp kabobs on the rack of an uncovered grill directly over medium coals for 10 to 12 minutes or until shrimp are opaque, turning once halfway through grilling. (Or, broil on the unheated rack of a broiler pan about 4 inches from the heat for 10 to 12 minutes, turning once halfway through broiling.) **FOUR** To serve, heat the reserved ¼ cup marinade. Spoon over shrimp and sprinkle with toasted coconut. If desired, serve over hot rice.

Hoisin and Citrus Shrimp Sauté

Sweet, spicy hoisin sauce joins with orange juice to create a perfectly balanced sauce for this savory shrimp and spinach sauté. If you like a spicier taste, sprinkle it with crushed red pepper before serving.

Exchanges: 1 Vegetable, 1 Starch, 1 Lean Meat, ½ Fat

Nutrition Facts per serving: 306 cal., 9 g total fat (1 g sat. fat), 129 mg chol., 372 mg sodium, 34 g carbo., 1 g fiber, 20 g pro.
Daily Values: 13% vit. A, 48% vit. C, 7% calcium, 18% iron

12	ounces fresh or frozen large shrimp in shells
2	tablespoons cooking oil
2	cloves garlic, minced
1	medium red sweet pepper, cut into thin strips
⅓	cup orange juice
3	tablespoons hoisin sauce
1½	cups shredded fresh spinach
2	cups hot cooked rice

Start to Finish: 25 minutes
Makes 4 servings

ONE Thaw shrimp, if frozen. Peel and devein shrimp. Rinse shrimp; pat dry with paper towels. Set aside. **TWO** In a large skillet heat 1 tablespoon of the oil over medium-high heat. Add garlic; cook and stir for 15 seconds. Add red sweet pepper; cook and stir about 3 minutes or until crisp-tender. Remove from skillet. **THREE** Add the remaining 1 tablespoon oil to skillet. Add the shrimp. Cook and stir about 3 minutes or until shrimp are opaque. Remove from skillet. Add orange juice and hoisin sauce. Bring to boiling; reduce heat. Simmer, uncovered, about 1 minute or until slightly thickened. Return shrimp and sweet pepper to skillet. Add the spinach; toss just until combined. **FOUR** To serve, spoon the shrimp mixture over hot cooked rice.

Buying Fish and Shellfish

You don't need to enjoy fishing to spot good quality fish and shellfish. Here are a few tips for buying the freshest catch of the day:
Look for fish with clear, bright bulging eyes; shiny, tight skin; red gills that aren't slippery; and flesh that feels firm and elastic. Fillets and steaks should be moist and have clean-cut edges. Avoid fish with a strong fishy odor; dull, bloody, or sunken eyes; and faded skin and gill color. Fresh shrimp should be moist and firm, have translucent flesh, and smell fresh. An ammonia smell and blackened edges or spots on the shells indicate poor quality shrimp. When selecting scallops, look for firm, sweet smelling scallops that are free of cloudy liquid. Spoiled scallops have a strong sulfur odor.

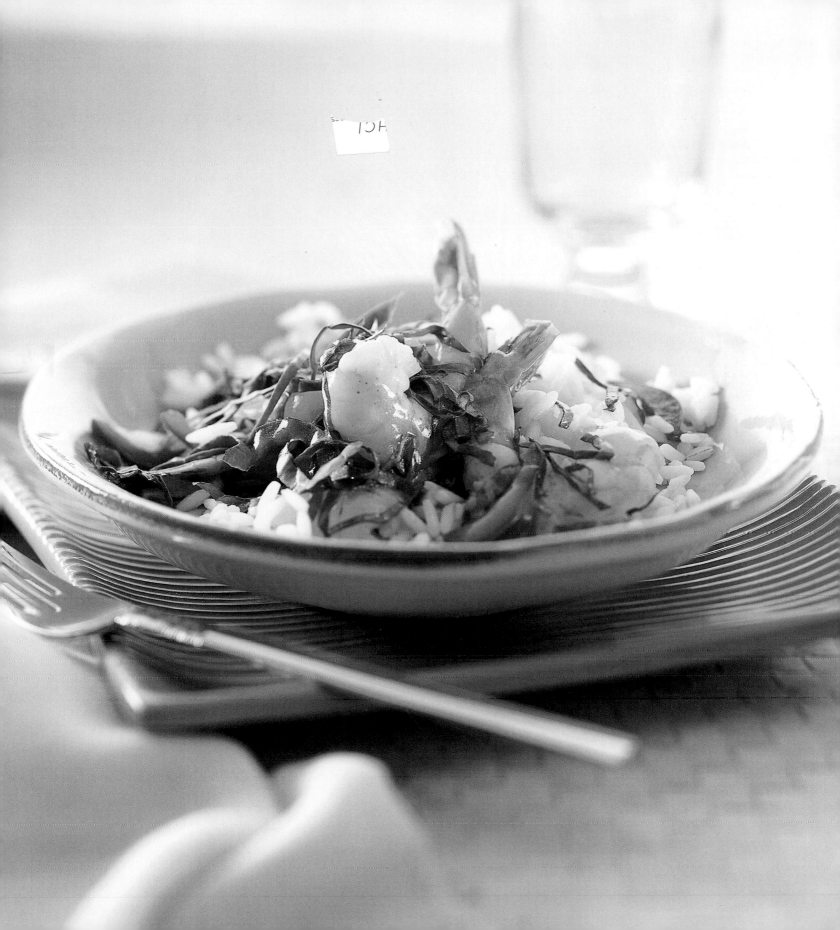

Moroccan Bouillabaisse

An aromatic blend of cumin, cinnamon, and ground red pepper scents your kitchen as this tasty seafood stew cooks on your stove. Discard any mussels that do not open after cooking.

Exchanges: 1 Starch, 1 Lean Meat

Nutrition Facts per serving: 187 cal., 6 g total fat (1 g sat. fat), 116 mg chol., 503 mg sodium, 12 g carbo., 1 g fiber, 23 g pro.
Daily Values: 10% vit. A, 30% vit. C, 33% iron

8 ounces fresh or frozen shrimp in shells

8 ounces fresh or frozen scallops

8 ounces fresh mussels in shells (8 to 12 mussels)

1 cup finely chopped onion

4 cloves garlic, minced

1 tablespoon olive oil

1 teaspoon ground cumin

1/2 teaspoon ground cinnamon

1/4 teaspoon ground red pepper

1 cup fish or vegetable broth

1 cup finely chopped tomatoes

1/4 teaspoon salt

1/8 teaspoon ground saffron

Hot cooked couscous

Prep: 30 minutes
Soak: 45 minutes
Cook: 5 minutes
Makes 4 servings

ONE Thaw shrimp and scallops, if frozen. Peel and devein shrimp. Rinse shrimp and scallops; pat dry with paper towels. Halve any large scallops. Scrub mussels under cold running water; remove beards. Combine 2 cups water and 3 tablespoons salt; add mussels and soak for 15 minutes. Drain and rinse mussels. Discard water. Repeat twice. **TWO** In a large saucepan cook onion and garlic in hot oil until onion is tender. Add cumin, cinnamon, and red pepper; cook and stir for 1 minute. Stir in broth, tomatoes, the 1/4 teaspoon salt, and the saffron. **THREE** Bring to boiling. Add shrimp, scallops, and mussels. Return to boiling; reduce heat. Simmer, covered, about 5 minutes or until the mussel shells open and the mussels are thoroughly cooked. **FOUR** To serve, divide the hot couscous among 4 shallow bowls. Ladle the seafood mixture over couscous.

Shrimp Gazpacho

Pack this invigorating cold soup of garden-ripe tomatoes, fresh cucumber, and succulent shrimp in an insulated container and head to the park. Grab a loaf of crusty bread and a bottle of wine to complete the picnic.

Exchanges: 2 Vegetable, ½ Lean Meat

Nutrition Facts per serving: 141 cal., 6 g total fat (1 g sat. fat), 74 mg chol., 154 mg sodium, 15 g carbo., 4 g fiber, 11 g pro.
Daily Values: 22% vit. A, 121% vit. C, 3% calcium, 37% iron

8	ripe medium tomatoes, peeled (if desired) and chopped
1	medium cucumber, chopped
1	medium green or red sweet pepper, chopped
¾	cup low-sodium vegetable juice
½	cup clam juice
¼	cup chopped onion
3	tablespoons red wine vinegar
2	tablespoons snipped fresh cilantro
2	tablespoons olive oil
1	clove garlic, minced
¼	teaspoon ground cumin
1	8-ounce package frozen peeled, cooked shrimp, thawed
	Fat-free dairy sour cream (optional)

Prep: 30 minutes
Chill: 4 hours
Makes 6 servings

ONE In a large bowl combine the tomatoes, cucumber, sweet pepper, vegetable juice, clam juice, onion, vinegar, cilantro, olive oil, garlic, and cumin. Stir in shrimp. **TWO** Cover and refrigerate for 4 to 24 hours to blend flavors. To serve, ladle into soup bowls. If desired, top each serving with sour cream.

Cholesterol and Shrimp

Three ounces of shrimp contains 129 mg cholesterol. That may seem high compared to chicken, which only provides 73 mg cholesterol per 3-ounce serving. But shrimp has some great attributes too. It's low in calories, saturated fat, and fat. So go ahead and satisfy your craving—just watch your total cholesterol intake from all foods.

seven.meatless main dishes

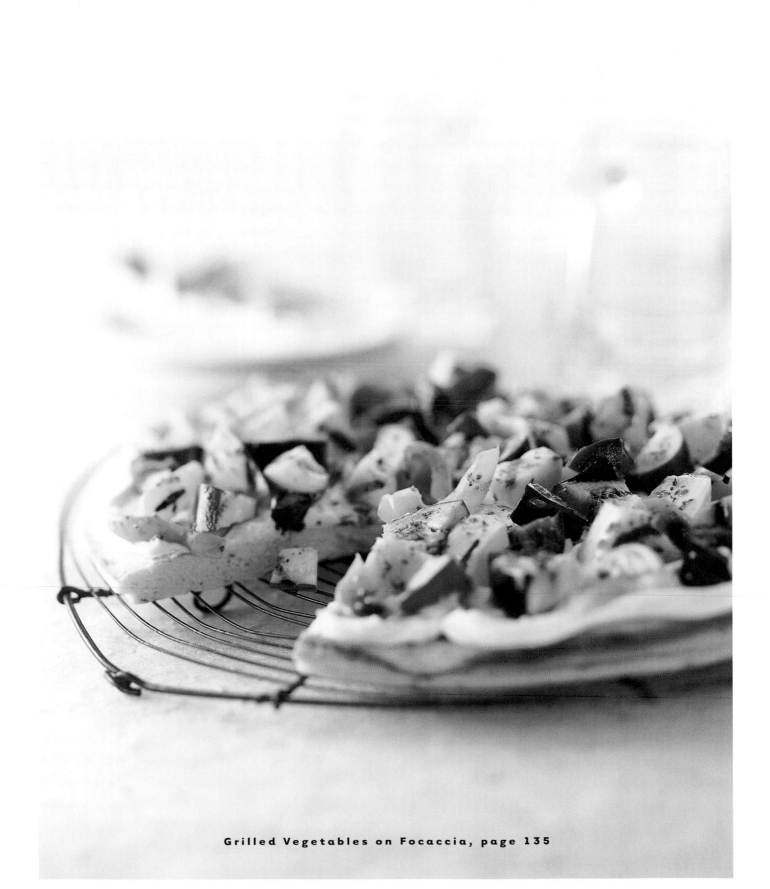

Grilled Vegetables on Focaccia, page 135

Sweet Bean Pilaf

Green soybeans, called edamame or sweet beans, are specially grown soybeans that are harvested when the seeds are immature. The nutty tasting beans are readily available in the freezer section of most supermarkets.

Exchanges: 2 Vegetable, 1 Fruit, 2½ Starch, ½ Fat

Nutrition Facts per serving: 348 cal., 9 g total fat (1 g sat. fat), 0 mg chol., 227 mg sodium, 56 g carbo., 19 g fiber, 16 g pro.
Daily Values: 50% vit. A, 113% vit. C, 18% calcium, 24% iron

1	medium onion, chopped
2	cloves garlic, minced
1	tablespoon olive oil
1	cup bulgur
1	cup frozen green or sweet soybeans (edamame)
1	cup orange juice
1	cup chicken or vegetable broth
1	medium carrot, cut into thin bite-size strips
1	stalk celery, bias-sliced
2	oranges, peeled and sectioned
⅓	cup dried tart cherries or raisins

Prep: 15 minutes
Cook: 10 minutes
Makes 4 servings

ONE In a large saucepan cook onion and garlic in hot oil until onion is tender. Stir in bulgur, soybeans, orange juice, broth, carrot, and celery. **TWO** Bring to boiling; reduce heat. Simmer, covered, for 10 to 12 minutes or until soybeans are tender and liquid is absorbed. Stir in oranges and dried cherries.

Three-Cheese-Stuffed Shells

In this low-fat version of stuffed shells, tofu replaces some of the cheese, boosting the protein and lowering the fat content. A trio of cheeses and Italian herbs ensures hearty, family-pleasing flavor.

Exchanges: ½ Vegetable, 1 Starch, 1 Lean Meat

Nutrition Facts per serving: 257 cal., 8 g total fat (2 g sat. fat), 73 mg chol., 906 mg sodium, 30 g carbo., 2 g fiber, 17 g pro.
Daily Values: 21% vit. A, 38% vit. C, 22% calcium, 17% iron

12   dried jumbo pasta shells

8   ounces soft tofu (fresh bean curd)

1   beaten egg

½   cup light ricotta cheese

½   cup shredded mozzarella cheese

¼   cup finely shredded Parmesan cheese

2   tablespoons snipped fresh parsley

½   teaspoon dried oregano, crushed

⅛   teaspoon black pepper

1   14½-ounce can Italian-style stewed tomatoes, undrained and cut up

1   8-ounce can tomato sauce

Finely shredded Parmesan cheese (optional)

Snipped fresh parsley (optional)

Prep: 25 minutes
Bake: 25 minutes
Makes 4 servings

ONE Cook pasta according to package directions; drain. Spread pasta shells in a single layer on a piece of greased foil to cool completely. **TWO** Meanwhile, for filling, in a medium bowl mash tofu with a fork. Stir in egg, ricotta cheese, mozzarella cheese, Parmesan cheese, parsley, oregano, and pepper. Spoon a scant ¼ cup filling into each cooked pasta shell. Arrange filled shells in a 2-quart square baking dish. **THREE** Combine the tomatoes and tomato sauce; pour over shells in baking dish. Bake, covered, in a 350° oven for 15 minutes. Bake, uncovered, for 10 to 15 minutes more or until heated through. If desired, sprinkle with additional Parmesan cheese and parsley.

Tofu 101

Tofu, sometimes called soybean curd or bean curd, is made by adding calcium to soy milk until it curdles. Much like cheese, the curds are then strained and pressed into cubes of varying firmness, depending on how much liquid is pressed out. When using tofu, match the firmness to the recipe. Soft or silken varieties blend into creamy consistencies for dips and sauces. Medium and firm tofu are best crumbled in casseroles, soups, salads, burgers, stuffings, and cheesecakes. Use the firmest tofus for stir-frying and grilling.

Fried Tofu and Vegetables

Crisp, cornmeal-crusted tofu tops a colorful mélange of sweet peppers and pea pods. To ensure a pleasing texture for fried tofu, be sure to purchase the extra-firm variety.

Exchanges: 1½ Vegetable, 1 Lean Meat, ½ Fat

Nutrition Facts per serving: 198 cal., 10 g total fat (1 g sat. fat), 0 mg chol., 410 mg sodium, 14 g carbo., 3 g fiber, 16 g pro.
Daily Values: 21% vit. A, 178% vit. C, 15% calcium, 63% iron

1	10½-ounce package light extra-firm tofu, well-drained
3	tablespoons reduced-sodium tamari sauce or soy sauce
8	green onions
8	ounces fresh pea pods (2 cups)
1	tablespoon toasted sesame oil
1	medium red sweet pepper, cut into thin strips
1	medium yellow sweet pepper, cut into thin strips
2	tablespoons cornmeal
1	tablespoon white or black sesame seeds, toasted* (optional)
	Fresh cilantro (optional)

Prep: 15 minutes
Stand: 1 hour
Cook: 9 minutes
Makes 4 servings

ONE Cut tofu crosswise into 8 slices. Arrange slices in a single layer on a large plate or shallow baking pan. Pour tamari sauce over tofu; turn slices to coat. Cover and let stand for 1 hour. **TWO** Meanwhile, trim ends of green onions, leaving 3 inches of white and light green parts. Cut green onions in half lengthwise, forming 16 strips. Trim ends of pea pods and remove strings; cut pea pods in half lengthwise. **THREE** Pour sesame oil into a 12-inch nonstick skillet. Preheat over medium-high heat. Stir-fry red and yellow peppers in hot oil for 1 minute. Add green onions and pea pods. Stir-fry for 2 to 3 minutes more or until vegetables are crisp-tender. Remove skillet from heat. Drain tofu, reserving tamari sauce. Stir the tamari sauce into cooked vegetables. Transfer to a serving platter; cover and keep warm. **FOUR** Carefully dip the tofu slices in cornmeal to lightly coat both sides. In the same skillet cook tofu about 6 minutes or until crisp and heated through, gently turning once. **FIVE** For each serving, place a tofu slice on a dinner plate. Top with cooked vegetables and another slice of tofu. If desired, sprinkle with sesame seeds and garnish with fresh cilantro sprigs. Serve immediately.

***Note:** To toast sesame seeds, in a nonstick skillet cook and stir sesame seeds over medium heat about 1 minute or just until golden brown. Watch closely so the seeds don't burn. Remove from heat and transfer to a bowl to cool completely.*

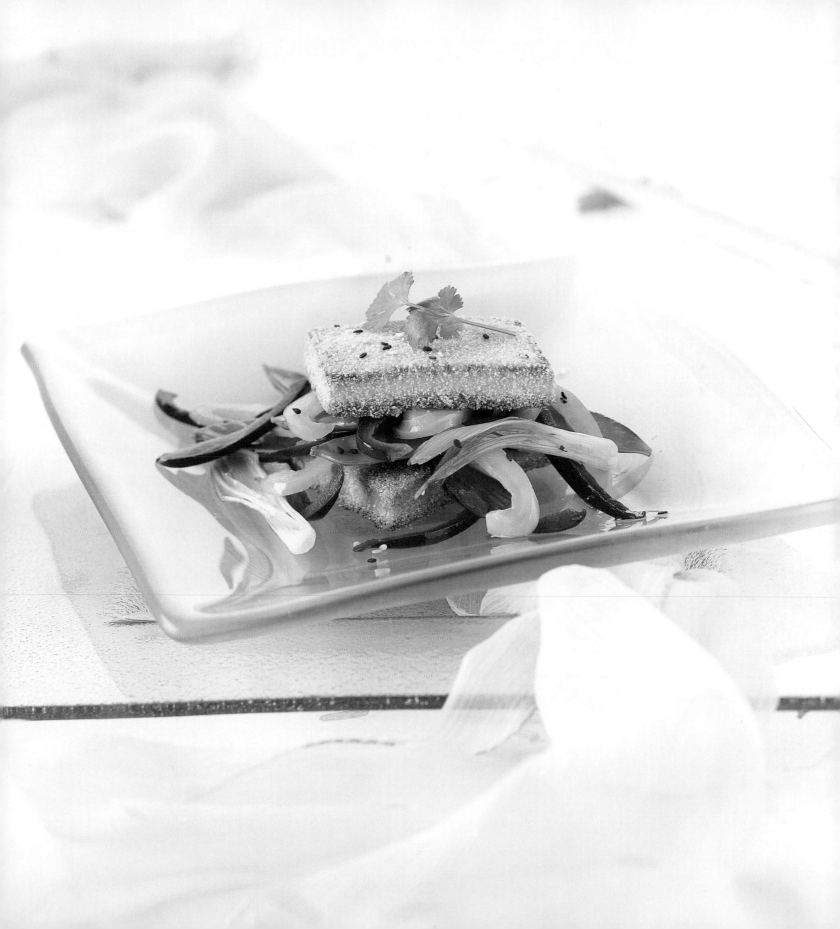

Herb and Pepper Lentil Stew

Fresh thyme and crushed red pepper mingle with the scent of seared onions in this high-fiber lentil stew. Just one serving provides almost half your daily fiber needs.

Exchanges: 1 Vegetable, 1 Starch, 1 Lean Meat

Nutrition Facts per serving: 241 cal., 4 g total fat (1 g sat. fat), 0 mg chol., 609 mg sodium, 39 g carbo., 10 g fiber, 15 g pro.
Daily Values: 4% vit. A, 41% vit. C, 6% calcium, 18% iron

1	tablespoon cooking oil
2	medium onions, quartered
1	medium green sweet pepper, cut into ½-inch rings
1	tablespoon snipped fresh thyme or 1 teaspoon dried thyme, crushed
¼	teaspoon crushed red pepper
5	cups water
1¼	cups dry red lentils,* rinsed and drained
1	teaspoon salt

Start to Finish: 35 minutes
Makes 4 servings

ONE In a Dutch oven heat oil over medium-high heat. Add onions; cook about 8 minutes or until browned, stirring occasionally. Add green pepper, thyme, and crushed red pepper. Cook and stir for 2 minutes. **TWO** Add the water, 1 cup of the lentils, and the salt. Bring to boiling; reduce heat. Simmer, uncovered, for 15 minutes. **THREE** Stir in the remaining ¼ cup lentils. Simmer, uncovered, for 4 minutes more.

__Note:__ Brown or green lentils can be substituted for the red lentils. Prepare Herb and Pepper Lentil Stew as directed, except add all of the lentils with the water. Bring to boiling; reduce heat. Simmer, covered, for 25 minutes. Simmer, uncovered, for 5 minutes more.

Lentil and Veggie Tostadas

Delve into these South-of-the-border tostadas for layers of cilantro- and cumin-spiked lentils, fresh veggies, and Monterey Jack cheese. Ready in 25 minutes, they're sure to become a family favorite.

Exchanges: ½ Milk, 1 Vegetable, 1 Starch, ½ Lean Meat

Nutrition Facts per serving: 288 cal., 11 g total fat (5 g sat. fat), 20 mg chol., 497 mg sodium, 34 g carbo., 7 g fiber, 16 g pro.
Daily Values: 24% vit. A, 68% vit. C, 18% calcium, 19% iron

1¾ cups water

¾ cup dry red lentils, rinsed and drained

¼ cup chopped onion

1 to 2 tablespoons snipped fresh cilantro

1 clove garlic, minced

½ teaspoon salt

½ teaspoon ground cumin

4 tostada shells

2 cups chopped fresh vegetables (such as broccoli, tomato, zucchini, and/or yellow summer squash)

¾ cup shredded Monterey Jack cheese (3 ounces)

Start to Finish: 25 minutes
Makes 4 servings

ONE In a medium saucepan stir together water, lentils, onion, cilantro, garlic, salt, and cumin. Bring to boiling; reduce heat. Simmer, covered, for 12 to 15 minutes or until lentils are tender and most of the liquid is absorbed. Use a fork to mash the cooked lentils.

TWO Spread the lentil mixture on tostada shells; top with the vegetables and cheese. Place on a large baking sheet. Broil tostadas 3 to 4 inches from the heat about 2 minutes or until cheese is melted.

Fiber Facts

Roughage, bulk, nature's little scrubbing brush—however you choose to describe it, fiber can be a great aid in your quest to lose weight. Fiber, the carbohydrates that cannot be digested by your body, can help make you feel full longer between meals. Strive to include between 25 and 35 grams of dietary fiber in your daily meal plan. To help boost your fiber intake, include fruit with edible skins, raw vegetables with edible skins and seeds, whole-grain breads and cereals, brown rice, bulgur, cooked or canned beans, and other legumes.

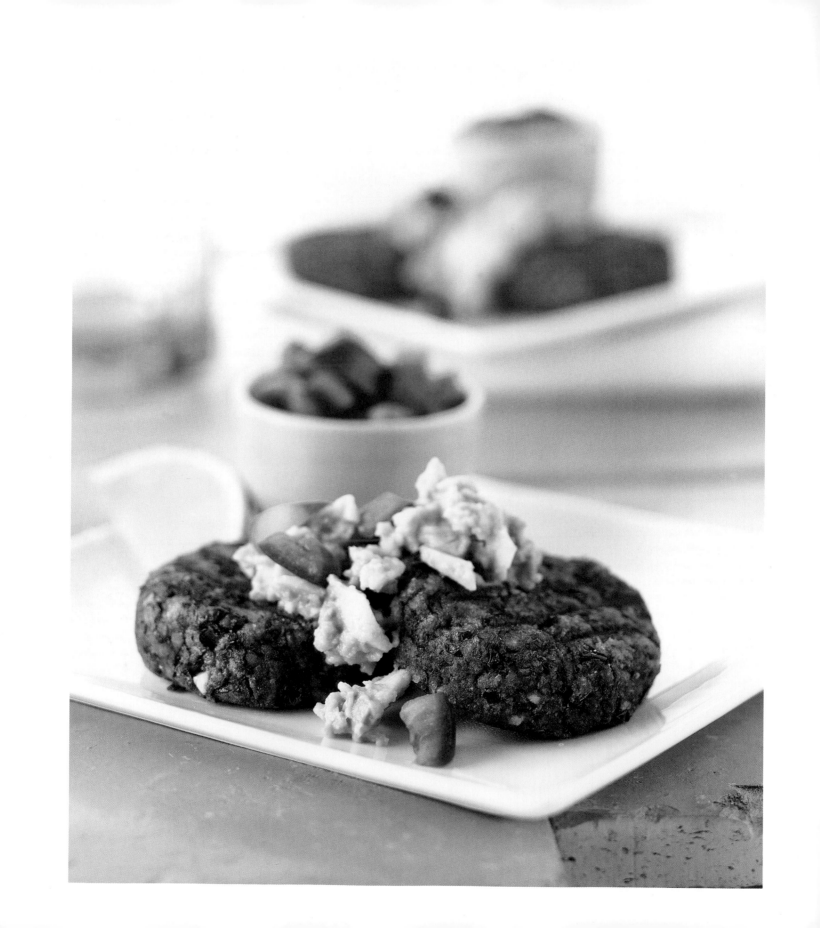

Southwestern Black Bean Cakes with Guacamole

Fire up the grill for great vegetarian fare. Spunky chipotle peppers team with pungent cumin in these black bean burgers.

Exchanges: ½ Vegetable, 1½ Starch, ½ Lean Meat

Nutrition Facts per serving: 178 cal., 7 g total fat (1 g sat. fat), 53 mg chol., 487 mg sodium, 25 g carbo., 9 g fiber, 11 g pro.
Daily Values: 9% vit. A, 12% vit. C, 7% calcium, 16% iron

½ of a medium avocado, seeded and peeled

1 tablespoon lime juice

2 slices whole wheat bread, torn

3 tablespoons fresh cilantro leaves

2 cloves garlic

1 15-ounce can black beans, rinsed and drained

1 canned chipotle pepper in adobo sauce

1 to 2 teaspoons adobo sauce

1 teaspoon ground cumin

1 egg

1 small plum tomato, chopped

Lime wedges (optional)

Prep: 20 minutes
Grill: 8 minutes
Makes 4 servings

ONE For guacamole, in a small bowl mash avocado. Stir in lime juice; season to taste with salt and black pepper. Cover surface with plastic wrap and set aside until ready to serve. **TWO** Place torn bread in a food processor bowl or blender container. Cover and process or blend until bread resembles coarse crumbs. Transfer bread crumbs to a large bowl; set aside. **THREE** Place cilantro and garlic in the food processor bowl or blender container. Cover and process or blend until finely chopped. Add the beans, chipotle pepper, adobo sauce, and cumin. Cover and process or blend using on/off pulses until beans are coarsely chopped and mixture begins to pull away from side of container. Add bean mixture to bread crumbs in bowl. Add egg; mix well. Shape into eight ½-inch-thick patties. **FOUR** Grill patties on the lightly greased rack of an uncovered grill directly over medium coals for 8 to 10 minutes or until the patties are heated through, turning once halfway through grilling. Serve the patties with guacamole, tomato, and, if desired, lime wedges.

Provençale Vegetable Stew

Savor this herb-filled vegetable stew on chilly fall evenings. Loaded with Mediterranean-style vegetables—eggplant, zucchini, and tomato—it makes eating your five-a-day a snap.

Exchanges: 3 Vegetable, 1 Starch, ½ Fat

Nutrition Facts per serving: 261 cal., 11 g total fat (2 g sat. fat), 5 mg chol., 861 mg sodium, 39 g carbo., 8 g fiber, 12 g pro.
Daily Values: 6% vit. A, 22% vit. C, 12% calcium, 18% iron

2	tablespoons olive oil
4	½-inch slices baguette-style French bread
¼	cup grated Romano cheese
2	baby eggplants or 1 very small eggplant (about 8 ounces)
2	large zucchini and/or yellow summer squash, quartered lengthwise and sliced ½ inch thick
4	cloves garlic, minced
1	14½-ounce can vegetable or chicken broth
1	15-ounce can white kidney (cannellini) or Great Northern beans, rinsed and drained
1	large tomato, chopped
1	tablespoon snipped fresh basil
2	teaspoons snipped fresh rosemary or thyme
¼	teaspoon black pepper
1	tablespoon balsamic vinegar

Start to Finish: 35 minutes
Makes 4 servings

ONE For croutons, lightly brush 2 teaspoons of the olive oil over one side of bread slices. Sprinkle with 2 tablespoons of the cheese. Place bread on a baking sheet. Bake in a 400° oven for 8 to 9 minutes or until toasted. Set aside. **TWO** Meanwhile, if desired, peel eggplant. Cut eggplant into ¾-inch cubes (you should have about 2 cups). In a large saucepan heat the remaining 4 teaspoons oil over medium-high heat. Add eggplant, zucchini, and garlic. Cook and stir for 5 minutes. Add the broth. **THREE** Bring to boiling; reduce heat. Simmer, uncovered, for 5 minutes. Stir in the beans. Simmer, uncovered, for 2 to 3 minutes more or until vegetables are tender. Stir in tomato, basil, rosemary, and pepper. Heat through. Remove from heat; stir in vinegar. **FOUR** To serve, ladle the vegetable mixture into bowls. Top with croutons and sprinkle with the remaining 2 tablespoons cheese.

Grilled Vegetables on Focaccia

For this open-face sandwich, spread focaccia with goat cheese and top with grilled vegetables. Or use a thicker focaccia and split it horizontally. Fill the focaccia with the veggies and goat cheese (see photo, page 125).

Exchanges: ½ Milk, 1 Vegetable, 1 Starch

Nutrition Facts per serving: 161 cal., 5 g total fat (1 g sat. fat), 8 mg chol., 240 mg sodium, 24 g carbo., 3 g fiber, 7 g pro.
Daily Values: 25% vit. A, 54% vit. C, 11% calcium, 4% iron

3	tablespoons balsamic vinegar or red wine vinegar
2	tablespoons water
1	tablespoon olive oil
1	teaspoon dried oregano, crushed
1	large zucchini and/or yellow summer squash, halved crosswise and sliced
2	small red and/or orange sweet peppers, quartered lengthwise
1	small eggplant, cut crosswise into ½-inch slices
1	12-inch Italian flat bread (focaccia)
2	ounces soft goat cheese (chèvre)
2	ounces fat-free cream cheese

Prep: 20 minutes
Grill: 8 minutes
Makes 8 servings

ONE In a large bowl combine the vinegar, water, oil, and oregano. Add the zucchini, sweet peppers, and eggplant; toss to coat. Drain vegetables, discarding vinegar mixture. **TWO** Grill vegetables on the rack of an uncovered grill directly over medium-hot coals until lightly browned and tender, turning occasionally. (Allow 5 to 6 minutes for zucchini and 8 to 10 minutes for peppers and eggplant.) Coarsely chop the grilled vegetables. **THREE** In a small bowl combine the goat cheese and cream cheese. Spread the cheese mixture over the focaccia. Top with the grilled vegetables. To serve, cut into wedges.

Fantastic Focaccia

A little like a lightly topped pizza without the sauce, focaccia is a much-loved Italian flat bread from the coastal region of Liguria. Generally, you'll find the best focaccia at artisanal or Italian bakeries; however, your grocery store might make its own version. In the above recipe, a purchased thin Italian flat bread was used as the base for the grilled veggies and goat cheese.

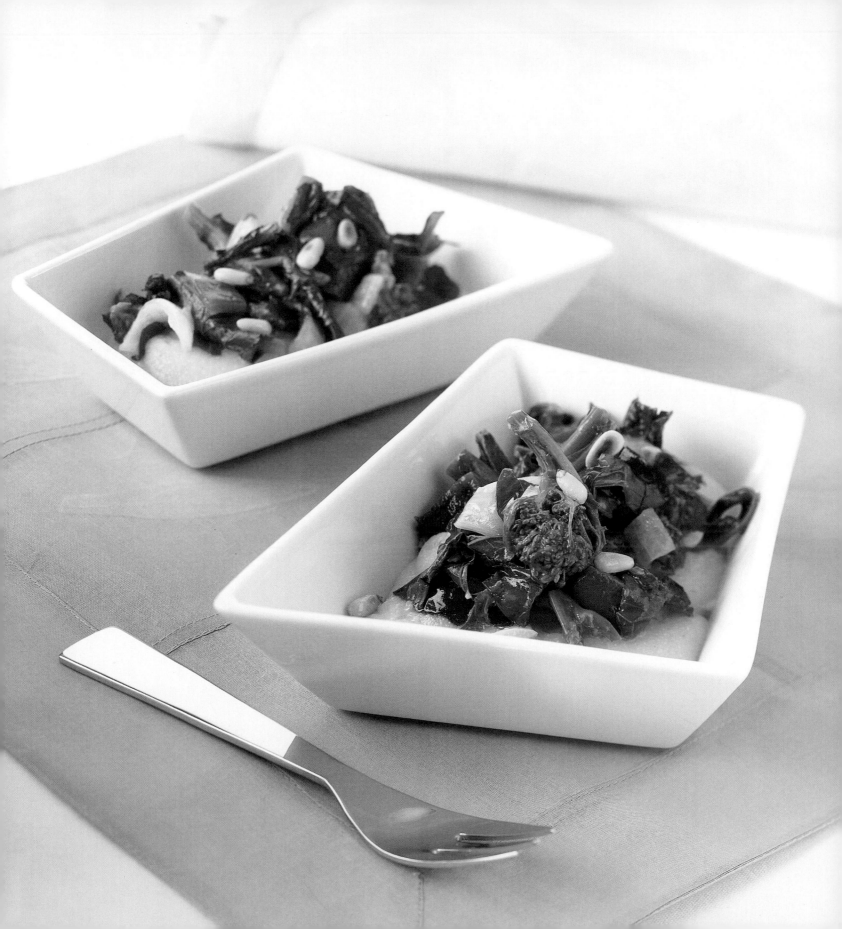

Broccoli Rabe over Polenta

Slightly bitter, crisp-tender broccoli rabe tastes superb when mixed with roasted sweet peppers and ladled over creamy polenta. If you can't find broccoli rabe, use broccoli flowerets or broccolini.

Exchanges: 2 Vegetable, 2 Starch, 1 Fat

Nutrition Facts per serving: 394 cal., 11 g total fat (1 g sat. fat), 0 mg chol., 256 mg sodium, 67 g carbo., 11 g fiber, 12 g pro.
Daily Values: 21% vit. A, 194% vit. C, 5% calcium, 18% iron

1	cup quick-cooking polenta mix
1	cup chopped sweet onion (such as Vidalia or Walla Walla)
4	teaspoons olive oil
3	cloves garlic, minced
1	pound broccoli rabe, coarsely chopped (about 7 cups), or 3 cups coarsely chopped broccoli flowerets
½	of a 7-ounce jar (½ cup) roasted red sweet peppers, rinsed, drained, and chopped
1	cup vegetable or chicken broth
1	tablespoon cornstarch
¼	cup pine nuts or slivered almonds, toasted (see tip, page 152)

Start to Finish: 30 minutes
Makes 4 servings

ONE Prepare polenta according to package directions. Cover and keep warm. **TWO** In a large skillet cook onion in hot oil over medium heat for 4 to 5 minutes or until tender. Add garlic; cook for 30 seconds. Add broccoli rabe. Cook, covered, about 3 minutes or just until tender. (If using broccoli flowerets, cook and stir for 3 to 4 minutes or until crisp-tender.) Stir in red peppers. **THREE** In a small bowl gradually stir broth into cornstarch; add to vegetable mixture. Cook and stir until thickened and bubbly. Cook and stir for 2 minutes more. **FOUR** To serve, divide the polenta among 4 serving dishes or dinner plates. Spoon the vegetable mixture over the cooked polenta. Sprinkle with toasted nuts.

Double Corn Tortilla Casserole

Spoon into this Southwestern-style strata and you'll find layers of corn tortillas, mozzarella cheese, and vegetables baked in a savory buttermilk custard.

Exchanges: 1 Vegetable, 2 Starch, 1 Meat

Nutrition Facts per serving: 281 cal., 8 g total fat (4 g sat. fat), 71 mg chol., 653 mg sodium, 36 g carbo., 0 g fiber, 18 g pro.
Daily Values: 15% vit. A, 51% vit. C, 36% calcium, 10% iron

Nonstick cooking spray

1½ cups frozen whole kernel corn

6 6-inch corn tortillas, torn into bite-size pieces

1 cup shredded reduced-fat mozzarella cheese (4 ounces)

½ cup sliced green onions

1 4-ounce can diced green chile peppers, drained

¼ cup finely chopped red sweet pepper

1 cup buttermilk

2 egg whites*

1 egg*

¼ teaspoon garlic salt

⅓ cup salsa

Prep: 20 minutes
Bake: 40 minutes
Stand: 5 minutes
Makes 4 servings

ONE Coat a 2-quart square baking dish with cooking spray; set aside. Cook corn according to package directions; drain well. Arrange half of the tortillas in the prepared baking dish. Top with half of the cheese, half of the corn, half of the green onions, half of the chile peppers, and half of the red sweet pepper. Repeat layers. **TWO** In a medium bowl beat together the buttermilk, egg whites, whole egg, and garlic salt. Pour over the tortilla mixture. **THREE** Bake, uncovered, in a 325° oven about 40 minutes or until a knife inserted near center comes out clean. Let stand 5 minutes before serving. Serve with salsa.

*Note: *You can substitute ½ cup refrigerated or frozen egg product, thawed, for the egg whites and whole egg.*

Broccoli Omelet Provençale

Steamed broccoli slaw scented with fresh oregano tops these easy-to-make oven omelets. Add a final touch of warmed pasta sauce for colorful, delicious dining.

Exchanges: 2 Vegetable, 1 Lean Meat, 1 Fat

Nutrition Facts per serving: 222 cal., 15 g total fat (6 g sat. fat), 439 mg chol., 454 mg sodium, 6 g carbo., 2 g fiber, 14 g pro.
Daily Values: 25% vit. A, 30% vit. C, 7% calcium, 11% iron

Nonstick cooking spray

12 eggs

¼ cup water

½ teaspoon garlic salt

⅛ teaspoon black pepper

3 cups packaged shredded broccoli (broccoli slaw mix)

2 tablespoons snipped fresh oregano or basil

1 10-ounce container refrigerated plum tomato pasta sauce, heated

Start to Finish: 20 minutes
Makes 6 servings

ONE Coat a 15×10×1-inch baking pan with cooking spray; set aside. For omelet, in a large bowl beat together the eggs, water, garlic salt, and pepper. Pour egg mixture into the prepared baking pan. Bake in a 400° oven about 7 minutes or until egg mixture is set, but still glossy and moist. **TWO** Meanwhile, place a steamer basket in a medium saucepan. Add water to just below bottom of steamer basket. Bring to boiling. Add the shredded broccoli. Steam, covered, for 2 to 3 minutes or until heated through. Stir in oregano. **THREE** To serve, cut omelet into six 5-inch squares. Transfer omelet squares to warm dinner plates. Spoon some of the broccoli mixture over half of each omelet square; fold other half of omelet over filling. Spoon the warm pasta sauce over omelets. Serve immediately.

Lycopene

Lycopene, one of the many carotenoids believed to reduce the risk of cancer, gives tomatoes, guava, watermelon, and pink grapefruit their red color. Because lycopene in tomatoes is more easily absorbed from processed items, food products such as tomato juice, tomato and pasta sauce, tomato paste, and catsup might have newfound respect.

Gazpacho Sandwich to Go

Juicy tomatoes, cucumber, onion, and mozzarella cheese redolent with mint vinaigrette pack the basil-lined bread. This sandwich is best when wrapped and chilled for several hours to let the flavors blend.

Exchanges: 1 Vegetable, 1½ Starch, 1 Milk

Nutrition Facts per serving: 237 cal., 8 g total fat (3 g sat. fat), 16 mg chol., 691 mg sodium, 29 g carbo., 3 g fiber, 12 g pro.
Daily Values: 17% vit. A, 42% vit. C, 24% calcium, 14% iron

½ of an 8-ounce loaf baguette-style French bread

¾ cup yellow pear-shaped, cherry, and/or grape tomatoes, quartered

¼ cup coarsely chopped cucumber

2 thin slices red onion, separated into rings

2 ounces fresh mozzarella cheese, cubed

1 tablespoon snipped fresh mint

1 tablespoon red wine vinegar

1 teaspoon olive oil

¼ teaspoon salt

⅛ teaspoon white pepper

½ cup fresh basil leaves

Prep: 20 minutes
Chill: 4 hours
Makes 2 servings

ONE Cut the bread in half crosswise. Slice each piece horizontally, making the bottom piece slightly larger than the top piece. Use a knife to carefully hollow out the bottom pieces, making ¼-inch shells. (Reserve the bread from centers for another use.) Set the bread shells aside. **TWO** In a medium bowl combine the tomatoes, cucumber, onion, mozzarella cheese, mint, vinegar, oil, salt, and white pepper. Line the bottoms of the bread shells with fresh basil leaves. Fill the shells with tomato mixture. Replace tops of bread. Wrap each sandwich in plastic wrap. Refrigerate at least 4 hours or overnight.

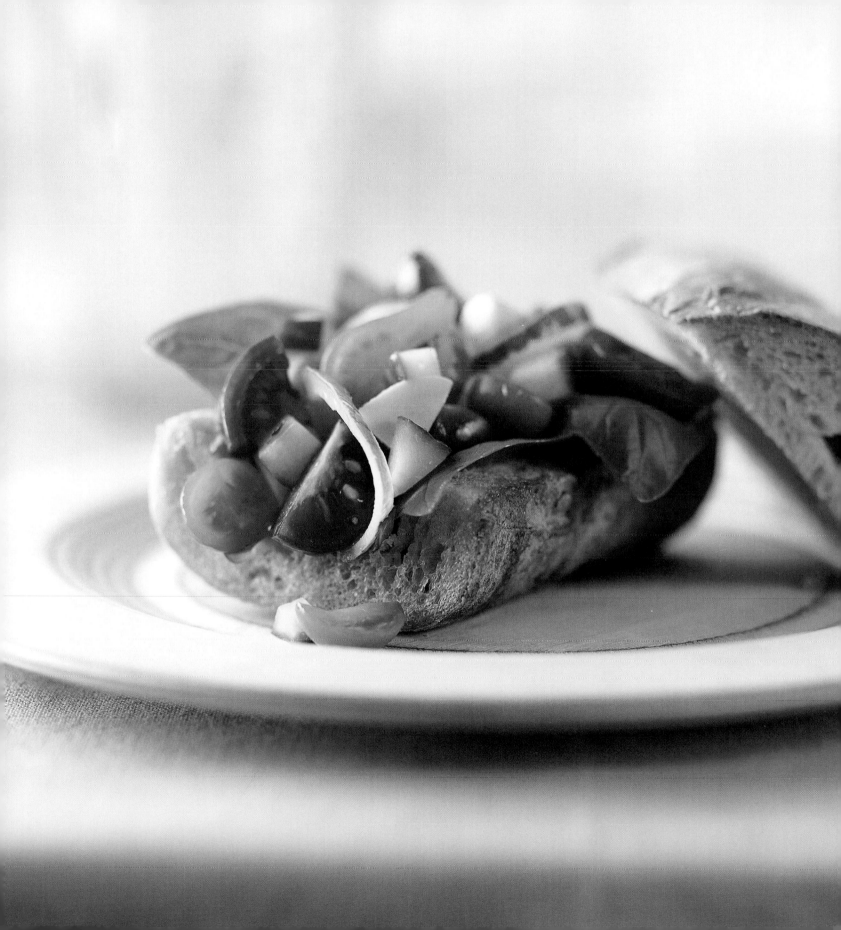

eight.sides

Lemon-Marinated Vegetables, page 145

Snow Peas and Tomatoes

Fresh, crisp snow peas star with plump, juicy grape tomatoes in this teriyaki- and sesame-seasoned side dish. If you want to add a little more pizzazz, use a combination of yellow and red cherry tomatoes.

Exchanges: 1 Vegetable, ½ Fat

Nutrition Facts per serving: 63 cal., 2 g total fat (o g sat. fat), o mg chol., 120 mg sodium, 8 g carbo., 2 g fiber, 3 g pro.
Daily Values: 3% vit. A, 41% vit. C, 5% calcium, 11% iron

2	teaspoons peanut oil
¼	teaspoon toasted sesame oil
1	large shallot, sliced
6	cups fresh pea pods, strings removed
1	tablespoon teriyaki sauce
½	cup grape or cherry tomatoes, halved
2	teaspoons sesame seeds, toasted*

Start to Finish: 15 minutes
Makes 6 servings

__ONE__ In a 12-inch skillet heat peanut oil and sesame oil over medium heat. Add shallot; cook until tender. Add the pea pods and teriyaki sauce. Cook and stir for 2 to 3 minutes or until pea pods are crisp-tender. Gently stir in tomatoes; cook for 1 minute more. __TWO__ Transfer the vegetable mixture to a serving bowl. Sprinkle with sesame seeds.

*Note: *To toast sesame seeds, in a nonstick skillet cook and stir sesame seeds over medium heat about 1 minute or just until golden brown. Watch closely so the seeds don't burn. Remove from heat and transfer to a bowl to cool completely.*

Lemon-Marinated Vegetables

With lively seasonings and vibrant colors, these vegetables brighten up the menu. Choose any combination of veggies you like, but cut any large ones into pieces the size of baby vegetables (see photo, page 143).

Exchanges: 2 Vegetable, ½ Fat

Nutrition Facts per serving: 59 cal., 2 g total fat (0 g sat. fat), 0 mg chol., 43 mg sodium, 9 g carbo., 3 g fiber, 2 g pro.
Daily Values: 88% vit. A, 36% vit. C, 3% calcium, 7% iron

½ teaspoon finely shredded lemon peel

2 tablespoons lemon juice

2 tablespoons water

1 tablespoon olive oil

2 teaspoons snipped fresh basil or oregano

1 teaspoon Dijon-style mustard

1 clove garlic, minced

2 pounds whole tiny vegetables (such as carrots, zucchini, and/or yellow summer squash) and/or cut-up pattypan squash

8 ounces sugar snap peas, trimmed

12 cherry tomatoes

Prep: 20 minutes
Chill: 2 hours
Makes 8 servings

ONE For dressing, in a screw-top jar combine lemon peel, lemon juice, water, olive oil, basil, mustard, and garlic. Set aside. **TWO** In a covered large saucepan cook the 2 pounds vegetables in a small amount of boiling water for 3 minutes. Add sugar snap peas. Cook, covered, for 2 to 3 minutes more or until vegetables are crisp-tender; drain. Rinse with cold water; drain again. **THREE** In a large bowl combine the cooked vegetables and tomatoes. Shake dressing. Pour over vegetables; toss gently to coat. Cover and refrigerate at least 2 hours or overnight.

Eat Your Veggies

Your mother was right—vegetables are good for you! Eating 3 to 5 servings per day helps meet nutrient goals for fiber, vitamins A and C, folate, iron, and magnesium. It's easy to meet these minimum requirements when you consider each of the following equals a serving:

1 cup raw leafy vegetables, such as spinach, cabbage, or lettuce

½ cup cooked or raw chopped vegetables, such as carrots, green beans, or broccoli

¾ cup vegetable juice

Orange-Sauced Broccoli and Peppers
A powerhouse vegetable combination—broccoli and sweet peppers—helps maintain healthy skin and aids your immune system. Serve this colorful combo with grilled fish or pork chops.

Exchanges: 1 Vegetable, ½ Fat

Nutrition Facts per serving: 58 cal., 2 g total fat (0 g sat. fat), 0 mg chol., 82 mg sodium, 8 g carbo., 3 g fiber, 2 g pro.
Daily Values: 15% vit. A, 118% vit. C, 3% calcium, 4% iron

3½ cups broccoli flowerets

1 medium red and/or yellow sweet pepper, cut into bite-size pieces

1 tablespoon margarine or butter

2 tablespoons finely chopped onion

1 clove garlic, minced

1½ teaspoons cornstarch

⅔ cup orange juice

2 teaspoons Dijon-style mustard

Start to Finish: 20 minutes
Makes 6 servings

ONE In a medium saucepan cook broccoli and sweet pepper in a small amount of boiling, lightly salted water about 8 minutes or until broccoli is crisp-tender; drain. Cover and keep warm. **TWO** Meanwhile, for sauce, in a small saucepan melt margarine over medium heat. Add onion and garlic; cook until onion is tender. Stir in cornstarch. Add orange juice and mustard. Cook and stir until mixture is thickened and bubbly. Cook and stir for 2 minutes more. **THREE** Pour the sauce over the broccoli mixture; toss gently to coat.

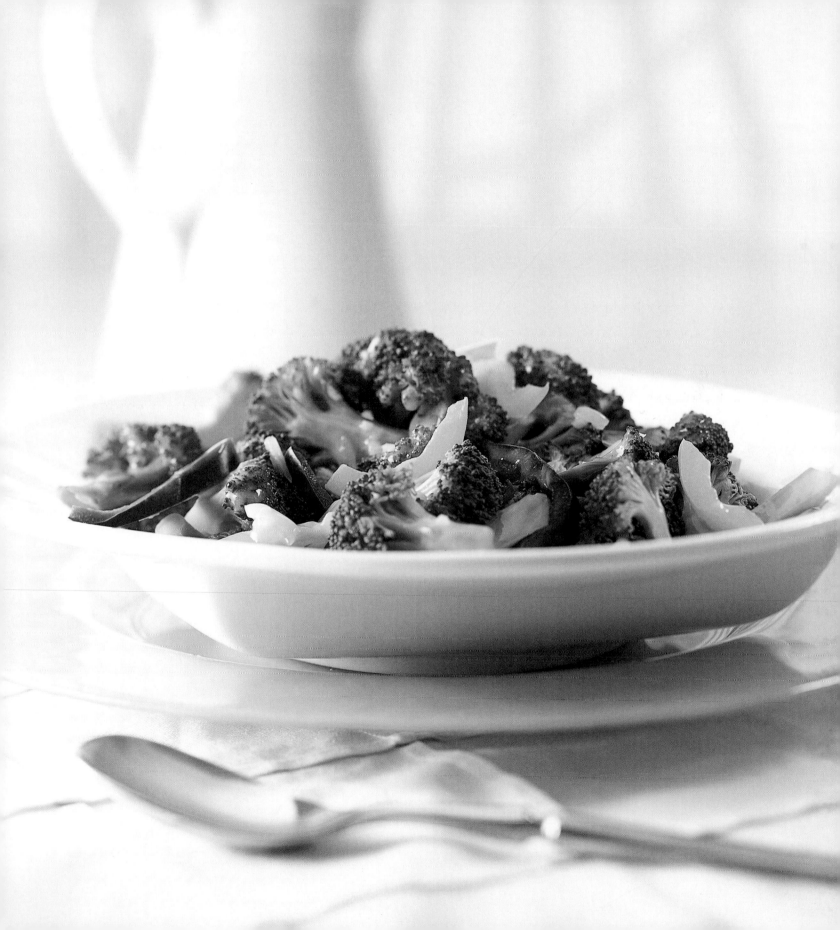

Braised and Seasoned Brussels Sprouts

A trio of seeds—mustard, cumin, and fennel—joins fresh ginger to add big, bold flavor to these cruciferous vegetables. Choose Brussels sprouts that are firm and vivid green in color.

Exchanges: 2 Vegetable, ½ Fat

Nutrition Facts per serving: 39 cal., 2 g total fat (0 g sat. fat), 0 mg chol., 240 mg sodium, 5 g carbo., 2 g fiber, 2 g pro.
Daily Values: 8% vit. A, 53% vit. C, 3% calcium, 7% iron

Nonstick cooking spray

½ teaspoon mustard seed

½ teaspoon cumin seed

½ teaspoon fennel seeds

8 ounces Brussels sprouts, halved (2 cups)

⅓ cup chicken or vegetable broth

2 teaspoons grated fresh ginger

¼ teaspoon salt

1 dried Thai red pepper, crushed, or ¼ teaspoon crushed red pepper

1 tablespoon coarsely chopped cashews or peanuts

2 teaspoons sherry vinegar or red wine vinegar

Prep: 15 minutes
Cook: 10 minutes
Makes 4 servings

ONE Lightly coat a medium saucepan with cooking spray. Heat saucepan over medium-high heat. Add the mustard seed, cumin seed, and fennel seeds. Cook and stir for 30 seconds. Add the Brussels sprouts, broth, ginger, salt, and red pepper. **TWO** Bring to boiling; reduce heat. Simmer, covered, for 10 to 12 minutes or until Brussels sprouts are tender, stirring occasionally. Stir in the nuts and vinegar.

Orange-Ginger Carrots

Orange juice, ginger, and honey add new zest to a bowl of cooked carrots. The piquant glaze would be equally delicious over chunks of cooked sweet potatoes or winter squash.

Exchanges: 2 Vegetable

Nutrition Facts per serving: 67 cal., 0 g total fat (0 g sat. fat), 0 mg chol., 70 mg sodium, 16 g carbo., 4 g fiber, 1 g pro.
Daily Values: 256% vit. A, 12% vit. C, 2% calcium, 4% iron

1	16-ounce package peeled baby carrots
2	tablespoons orange juice
1	tablespoon honey
½	teaspoon grated fresh ginger
1	tablespoon snipped fresh parsley
	Finely shredded orange peel (optional)

Start to Finish: 15 minutes
Makes 4 servings

ONE In a covered large saucepan cook the carrots in a small amount of boiling water for 3 to 5 minutes or until crisp-tender. Drain carrots well. **TWO** Meanwhile, in a small bowl stir together the orange juice, honey, and ginger. Drizzle over carrots; toss to coat. **THREE** To serve, transfer the carrots to a serving bowl. Sprinkle with parsley and, if desired, orange peel.

Eating Out

When dining out, do you let your best intentions go out the window? Good news! You don't need to stay home to eat healthy meals. Here's how.

Plan ahead: *Consider your whole day's eating plan and make your choices accordingly.*

Pick your restaurant wisely: *Choose a restaurant that has a variety of menu alternatives and offers specially prepared foods.*

Be hungry but not too hungry: *If you save all of your calories for an evening of dining out, you might be ravenous and apt to overeat.*

Choose your meal wisely: *Choose foods that have been prepared simply (steamed vegetables, broiled or baked meat, poultry, or fish). Watch portion sizes. Most restaurants serve twice the normal portion size. You might want to split an entrée with your dinner partner.*

Take it slow: *Pause frequently during the meal to be sure you are still hungry. (You can take any remaining food home for lunch!)*

Skip dessert: *No? If this is not an option for you, choose a fruit alternate or split a rich dessert with your dinner partner.*

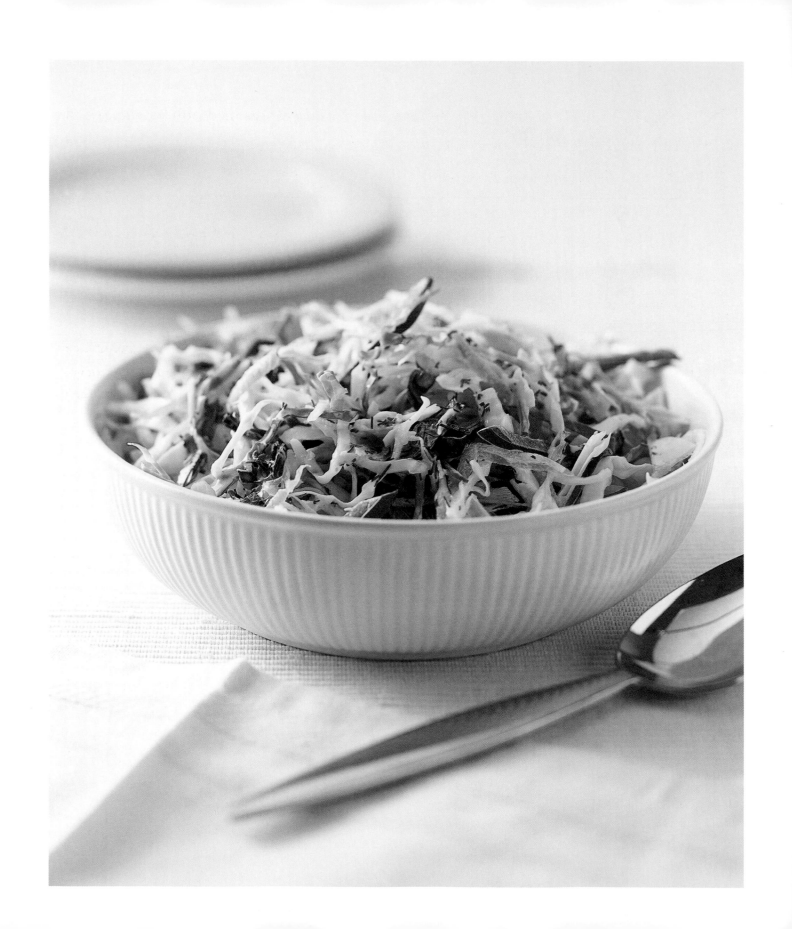

Coleslaw with a Twist

Red and green cabbage, seasoned with lime juice and fresh dillweed, bring new flavor to coleslaw. To prevent the red cabbage from coloring the coleslaw, rinse the shredded cabbage under cold water until the water runs clear.

Exchanges: 1 Vegetable, ½ Fat

Nutrition Facts per serving: 57 cal., 4 g total fat (1 g sat. fat), 3 mg chol., 146 mg sodium, 7 g carbo., 2 g fiber, 1 g pro.
Daily Values: 49% vit. A, 63% vit. C, 3% calcium, 2% iron

6	cups shredded green cabbage (1¼-pound head)
1	cup shredded red cabbage
1	medium carrot, shredded
½	of a small red sweet pepper, cut into thin bite-size strips
⅓	cup light mayonnaise dressing or salad dressing
2	tablespoons lime juice or lemon juice
1	tablespoon snipped fresh dill or 1 teaspoon dried dillweed (optional)
1	teaspoon sugar
¼	teaspoon salt
¼	teaspoon black pepper

Prep: 20 minutes
Chill: 2 hours
Makes 8 to 10 servings

ONE In a large bowl combine the green cabbage, red cabbage, carrot, and red sweet pepper. **TWO** For dressing, in a small bowl stir together the mayonnaise dressing, lime juice, dill (if desired), sugar, salt, and pepper. **THREE** Pour the dressing over cabbage mixture; toss to coat. (Mixture might appear dry at first, but will become moist as it chills.) Cover and refrigerate for 2 to 24 hours. Stir before serving.

Spinach-Apricot Salad
A little garlic and balsamic vinegar team up for an abundance of flavor in this wilted spinach salad. A handful of dried apricots adds a pleasing color and a touch of sweetness.

Exchanges: 1½ Vegetable, ½ Fruit, 1 Fat

Nutrition Facts per serving: 91 cal., 6 g total fat (1 g sat. fat), 0 mg chol., 146 mg sodium, 9 g carbo., 7 g fiber, 3 g pro.
Daily Values: 40% vit. A, 16% vit. C, 6% calcium, 27% iron

---

1   10-ounce package torn fresh baby spinach

⅓   cup dried apricots, snipped

1   tablespoon olive oil

1   clove garlic, thinly sliced or minced

4   teaspoons balsamic vinegar

2   tablespoons slivered almonds, toasted

Start to Finish: 20 minutes
Makes 4 servings

ONE If desired, remove stems from spinach. In a large bowl combine spinach and dried apricots. Set aside. **TWO** In a 12-inch skillet heat oil over medium heat. Add garlic; cook and stir until golden. Add the balsamic vinegar. Bring to boiling; remove from heat. **THREE** Add the spinach mixture. Toss mixture in skillet about 1 minute or just until spinach is wilted. **FOUR** Transfer the spinach mixture to a salad bowl. Season to taste with salt and black pepper. Sprinkle with almonds. Serve immediately.

Toasting Nuts

Toasting heightens the flavor of nuts, and it's simple to do. Spread nuts in a single layer in a shallow baking pan. Bake in a 350° oven for 5 to 10 minutes or until light golden brown, watching carefully and stirring once or twice so the nuts don't burn. Nuts can also be toasted in the microwave oven. Place nuts in a 2-cup measure. Microwave, uncovered, on 100 percent power (high), stirring after 2 minutes, then stirring every 30 seconds until light golden brown.

Fruit Salsa in a Big Way

Sweet, summer-fresh peaches, apricots, and cherries deftly balance the pungent flavors of lime juice, cilantro, and serrano peppers—making this salsa the perfect condiment for grilled chicken, turkey, or pork.

Exchanges: 1 Fruit

Nutrition Facts per serving: 75 cal., 0 g total fat (0 g sat. fat), 0 mg chol., 2 mg sodium, 19 g carbo., 3 g fiber, 1 g pro.
Daily Values: 10% vit. A, 24% vit. C, 1% calcium, 2% iron

3	medium peaches, peeled and cut into ¼- to ½-inch slices
3	small apricots, halved and pitted
8	ounces dark or light sweet cherries (such as Bing or Rainier), halved and pitted
4	ounces yellow pear-shaped tomatoes, halved, or 1 medium yellow tomato, cut into 1-inch pieces
2	to 3 fresh serrano peppers, seeded and finely chopped (see tip, below)
¼	cup lime juice
2	tablespoons snipped fresh cilantro
1	to 2 tablespoons sugar
	Lime wedges (optional)

Prep: 15 minutes
Chill: 30 minutes
Makes 10 servings

ONE In a large bowl combine the peaches, apricots, cherries, tomatoes, serrano peppers, lime juice, cilantro, and sugar. **TWO** Cover and refrigerate for at least 30 minutes or up to 12 hours. If desired, serve with lime wedges.

Handling Hot Peppers

Because fresh chile peppers, such as jalapeños and serranos, contain volatile oils that can burn your skin and eyes, avoid direct contact with them as much as possible. When working with chile peppers, wear plastic or rubber gloves. No gloves? Work with plastic bags over your hands. If you touch the chile pepper with your bare hands, wash them thoroughly with soap and water.

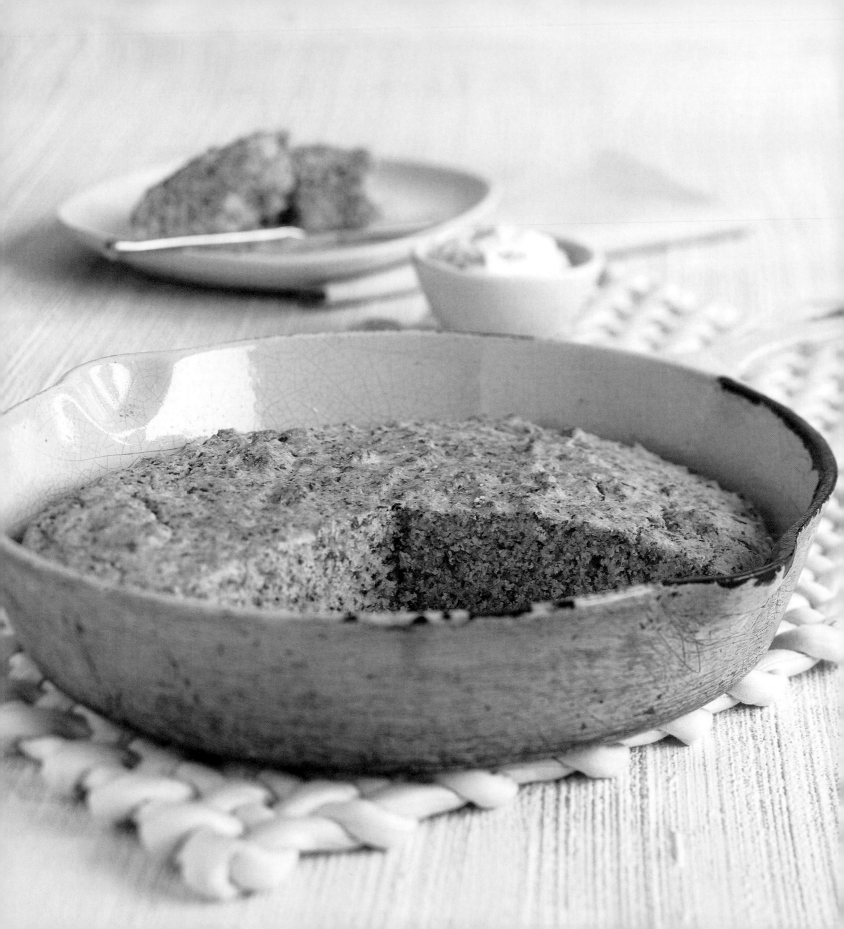

Flax Seed Corn Bread

Mild, nutty flax seed meal packs extra doses of calcium, iron, niacin, phosphorus, vitamin E, and omega-3 fatty acids into this simple loaf. Serve the corn bread warm from the oven with hearty winter soups.

Exchanges: 2 Starch, 1 Fat

Nutrition Facts per serving: 256 cal., 12 g total fat (2 g sat. fat), 54 mg chol., 482 mg sodium, 30 g carbo., 4 g fiber, 7 g pro.
Daily Values: 3% vit. A, 1% vit. C, 12% calcium, 12% iron

1	cup all-purpose flour
1	cup cornmeal
½	cup flax seed meal (see tip, below)
1	to 2 tablespoons flax seed
2	teaspoons baking powder
1½	teaspoons sugar
1	teaspoon salt
¼	teaspoon baking soda
2	beaten eggs
1	cup buttermilk
¼	cup olive oil
1	recipe Basil Butter (optional)

Prep: 15 minutes
Bake: 25 minutes
Makes 8 servings

ONE Place a well-greased 10-inch cast iron skillet in the oven while preheating oven to 375°. **TWO** Meanwhile, in a large bowl stir together flour, cornmeal, flax seed meal, flax seed, baking powder, sugar, salt, and baking soda. Set aside. **THREE** In a medium bowl combine eggs, buttermilk, and olive oil. Add the buttermilk mixture to the flour mixture. Stir just until moistened. Carefully spread the batter in the preheated skillet. **FOUR** Bake for 25 to 30 minutes or until golden brown and a wooden toothpick inserted in the center comes out clean. Cool slightly on a wire rack. If desired, serve the warm corn bread with Basil Butter.

Basil Butter:
In a small bowl stir together ⅓ cup butter, softened; 1 tablespoon finely snipped fresh basil or ¼ teaspoon dried basil, crushed; 1 clove garlic, minced; and ¼ teaspoon black pepper. Makes about ⅓ cup.

Flax Seed Meal
Ground flax seed provides more health benefits than whole flax seed because it's easier for the body to digest. Use a coffee grinder, blender, or food processor to grind the seeds. Use about ⅓ cup flax seed to make ½ cup meal. Because the ground seeds might become rancid, giving an off-flavor and taste, it's best to grind seeds as you need them. However, you can store ground seeds in an airtight, opaque container in the refrigerator for up to 3 months. Store whole seeds in an airtight container at room temperature up to 1 year.

Wheat and Oat Bread

Made with whole grains and embellished with a crunchy wheat-germ crust, this bread is an enticing accompaniment for garden-fresh salads or steaming bowls of soup.

Nonstick cooking spray

1¾ cups all-purpose flour

¾ cup whole wheat flour

½ cup regular rolled oats, toasted*

3 tablespoons toasted wheat germ

3 tablespoons sugar

2½ teaspoons baking powder

¼ teaspoon salt

1⅓ cups fat-free milk

¼ cup refrigerated or frozen egg product, thawed

2 tablespoons cooking oil

1 tablespoon toasted wheat germ

Prep: 20 minutes
Bake: 35 minutes
Makes 16 servings

ONE Coat the bottom and side of an 8×1½-inch round baking pan with cooking spray; set aside. **TWO** In a large bowl stir together the all-purpose flour, whole wheat flour, toasted oats, the 3 tablespoons wheat germ, the sugar, baking powder, and salt. In a medium bowl combine the milk, egg product, and oil. Add the milk mixture all at once to the flour mixture. Stir just until moistened (batter should be lumpy). Spread the batter into the prepared baking pan. Sprinkle with the 1 tablespoon wheat germ. **THREE** Bake in a 375° oven for 35 to 40 minutes or until golden brown and a wooden toothpick inserted near center comes out clean. Cool bread in pan on a wire rack for 10 minutes. Remove from pan. Serve warm.

*****Note:** *To toast rolled oats, place in a shallow baking pan. Bake in a 350° oven for 5 to 8 minutes or until oats are lightly browned, shaking pan once.*

Easy Herb Focaccia

The sprightly combination of onion and rosemary tops this quick-to-fix bread, conjuring images of Mediterranean sun and fun. A package of hot roll mix makes it easy for both novice and expert bakers.

Exchanges: 1 Starch

Nutrition Facts per serving: 88 cal., 2 g total fat (0 g sat. fat), 9 mg chol., 113 mg sodium, 15 g carbo., 0 g fiber, 3 g pro.
Daily Values: 3% iron

Nonstick cooking spray

1   16-ounce package hot roll mix

1   egg

2   tablespoons olive oil

2   teaspoons olive oil

⅔   cup finely chopped onion

1   teaspoon dried rosemary, crushed

Prep: 25 minutes
Rise: 30 minutes
Bake: 15 minutes
Makes 24 servings

ONE Coat a 15×10×1-inch baking pan or a 12- to 14-inch pizza pan with cooking spray; set aside. **TWO** Prepare the hot roll mix according to package directions for the basic dough, using the 1 egg and substituting the 2 tablespoons olive oil for the margarine. Knead dough; allow to rest as directed. If using the large baking pan, roll dough into a 15×10-inch rectangle and carefully transfer to the prepared pan. If using the pizza pan, roll dough into a 12-inch circle and carefully transfer to the prepared pan. **THREE** In a small saucepan heat the 2 teaspoons olive oil over medium heat. Add the onion and rosemary; cook until onion is tender. With your fingertips, press indentations every inch or so in dough. Top the dough evenly with onion mixture. Cover and let rise in a warm place until nearly double in size (about 30 minutes). **FOUR** Bake in a 375° oven for 15 to 20 minutes or until golden brown. Cool in pan on a wire rack for 10 minutes. Remove focaccia from pan; cool completely.

Parmesan and Pine Nut Focaccia:

Prepare Easy Herb Focaccia as directed, except omit the 2 teaspoons olive oil, the onion, and rosemary. Make the indentations, then brush the dough with a mixture of 1 egg white and 2 tablespoons water. Sprinkle with ¼ cup pine nuts, pressing lightly into dough. Sprinkle with 2 tablespoons grated Parmesan cheese. Bake as directed.
Nutrition Facts per serving: 95 cal., 3 g total fat (0 g sat. fat), 9 mg chol., 122 mg sodium, 15 g carbo., 0 g fiber, 4 g protein. Daily Values: 4% iron.

Oven-Roasted Autumn Vegetables

Roasting caramelizes the natural sugars in these vitamin-packed fall veggies, adding flavor without calories. A drizzle of walnut oil and balsamic vinegar further enriches this vegetable combo.

Exchanges: 1 Vegetable, 1½ Starch, ½ Fat

Nutrition Facts per serving: 198 cal., 7 g total fat (1 g sat. fat), 0 mg chol., 562 mg sodium, 31 g carbo., 11 g fiber, 4 g pro.
Daily Values: 109% vit. A, 41% vit. C, 5% calcium, 15% iron

1	fennel bulb, trimmed and cut into wedges
1	large sweet potato, peeled and cut into 1-inch cubes
8	ounces new red potatoes, quartered
4	large shallots, quartered
2	tablespoons walnut oil or olive oil
2	tablespoons balsamic vinegar
1	teaspoon coarse salt

Prep: 15 minutes
Roast: 30 minutes
Makes 4 to 6 servings

ONE In a large roasting pan toss together the fennel, sweet potato, red potatoes, shallots, oil, 1 tablespoon of the balsamic vinegar, and the salt. **TWO** Roast, uncovered, in a 425° oven for 30 to 35 minutes or until the vegetables are lightly browned and tender, stirring once or twice. **THREE** Transfer the roasted vegetables to a large serving bowl. Sprinkle with the remaining vinegar; toss gently to coat. Serve warm or at room temperature.

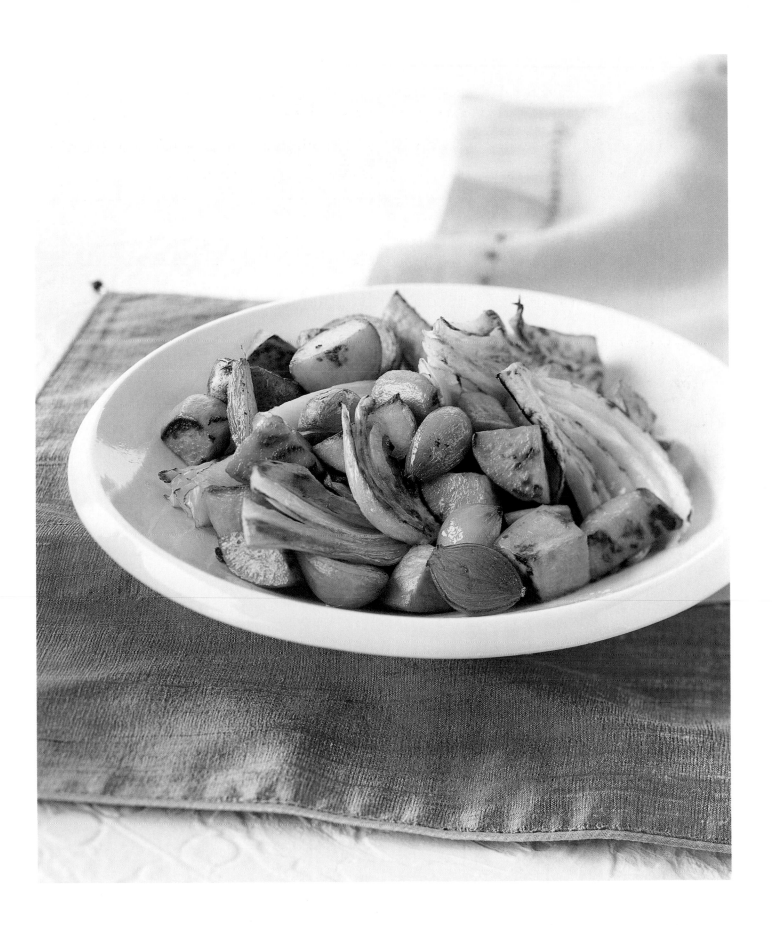

Lemon Prosciutto Potato Salad

Thin strips of prosciutto, a strongly flavored Italian ham, and delectable plum tomatoes set this potato salad apart from others. It makes enough to serve a crowd or to enjoy as leftovers the next day.

Exchanges: 1 Vegetable, 1 Starch, ½ Fat

Nutrition Facts per serving: 132 cal., 5 g total fat (1 g sat. fat), 51 mg chol., 411 mg sodium, 17 g carbo., 2 g fiber, 6 g pro.
Daily Values: 10% vit. A, 34% vit. C, 2% calcium, 7% iron

6	medium red potatoes (2 pounds), sliced ⅛ to ¼ inch thick
⅓	cup light mayonnaise dressing or salad dressing
3	cloves garlic, minced
1	teaspoon finely shredded lemon peel
½	teaspoon salt
¼	teaspoon black pepper
⅛	to ¼ teaspoon ground red pepper (optional)
4	plum tomatoes, cut lengthwise into wedges
3	ounces thinly sliced prosciutto, cut into thin strips
	Romaine lettuce leaves
2	hard-cooked eggs, chopped
	Snipped fresh parsley

Prep: 25 minutes
Chill: 2 hours
Makes 10 to 12 servings

ONE In a large saucepan cook potatoes in boiling, lightly salted water for 15 minutes or just until tender. Drain; cool slightly. **TWO** In a large bowl stir together the mayonnaise dressing, garlic, lemon peel, salt, black pepper, and, if desired, red pepper. Add the potatoes; toss gently to coat. Cover and refrigerate for 2 to 24 hours. **THREE** To serve, add the tomatoes and prosciutto to potato mixture; toss gently to combine. Line a serving bowl with romaine leaves. Spoon the potato mixture into the lettuce-lined bowl. Sprinkle with the chopped hard-cooked eggs and parsley.

Hearty Bulgur Pilaf

If you struggle to eat enough fiber and veggies, try this easy bulgur pilaf. With its pleasing, nutty flavor, bulgur is an excellent fiber source and provides a harmonious background flavor for the zucchini and carrots.

Exchanges: ½ Vegetable, 1 Starch

Nutrition Facts per serving: 78 cal., 1 g total fat (0 g sat. fat), 0 mg chol., 160 mg sodium, 17 g carbo., 5 g fiber, 3 g pro.
Daily Values: 40% vit. A, 2% vit. C, 1% calcium, 4% iron

1	14½-ounce can reduced-sodium chicken broth
1	medium zucchini, quartered lengthwise and sliced ½ inch thick
1	cup bulgur
2	medium carrots, cut into thin bite-size strips
½	cup chopped onion
2	tablespoons snipped fresh oregano or ½ teaspoon dried oregano, crushed
¼	teaspoon crushed red pepper
½	teaspoon finely shredded lemon peel

Start to Finish: 25 minutes
Makes 8 servings

ONE In a medium saucepan stir together the chicken broth, zucchini, bulgur, carrots, onion, dried oregano (if using), and crushed red pepper. **TWO** Bring to boiling; reduce heat. Simmer, covered, for 12 to 15 minutes or until bulgur is tender and broth is absorbed. Stir in the fresh oregano (if using) and lemon peel.

The Benefits of Bulgur

Bulgur is made from wheat kernels that have been steamed, dried, and crushed into small pieces. A ½-cup serving has 114 calories, less than half a gram of fat, and is a good source of complex carbohydrates and protein. You'll find bulgur next to the rice in your supermarket. It comes in three grain sizes: fine, medium, and coarse. Choose medium or coarse grain for the pilaf above.

Squash with Apples and Cranberries

Tart cranberries provide a pleasing contrast to sweet acorn squash and apple slices. If you prefer butternut or delicata squash, try those varieties instead of the acorn squash.

Exchanges: 1 Fruit, 1½ Starch

Nutrition Facts per serving: 207 cal., 3 g total fat (0 g sat. fat), 0 mg chol., 19 mg sodium, 48 g carbo., 6 g fiber, 3 g pro.
Daily Values: 141% vit. A, 46% vit. C, 7% calcium, 9% iron

---

2 acorn squash (2 to 2½ pounds total)

Nonstick cooking spray

1½ cups fresh or frozen cranberries

⅓ cup frozen apple juice concentrate, thawed

3 tablespoons brown sugar

1 teaspoon finely shredded orange peel

⅛ teaspoon ground cloves

2 medium tart apples (such as Granny Smith), peeled, cored, and cut into ½-inch slices

2 tablespoons maple-flavored syrup

2 tablespoons chopped pecans, toasted (see tip, page 152)

Prep: 10 minutes
Bake: 25 minutes
Makes 5 servings

ONE Cut squash crosswise into ½-inch slices. Remove seeds and strings. Lightly coat a 15×10×1-inch baking pan with cooking spray. Arrange squash in baking pan, overlapping slices if necessary. Bake, uncovered, in a 350° oven for 25 to 30 minutes or until squash is tender, turning once during baking. **TWO** Meanwhile, in a medium saucepan combine cranberries, apple juice concentrate, brown sugar, orange peel, and cloves. Bring to boiling; reduce heat. Simmer, uncovered, about 5 minutes or until slightly thickened. Stir in apples. Simmer, covered, about 7 minutes more or just until apples are tender, stirring occasionally. Remove from heat. Stir in syrup. **THREE** To serve, arrange squash slices on plate. Spoon the apple mixture over the squash pieces. Sprinkle with toasted pecans.

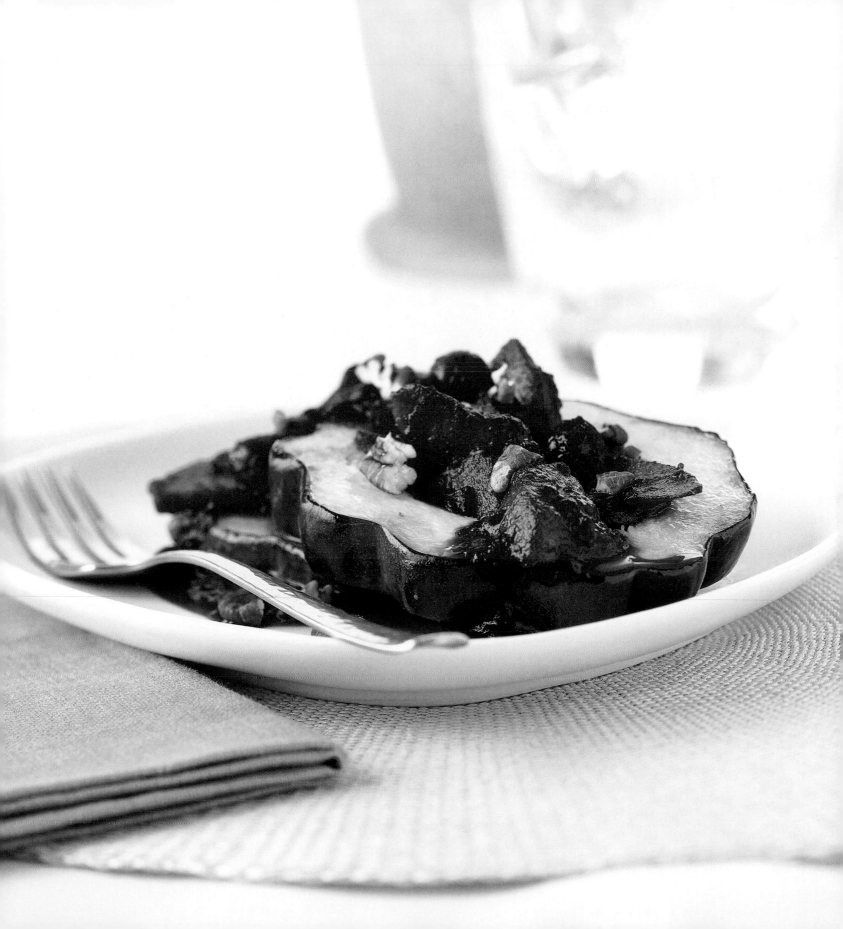

nine.desserts

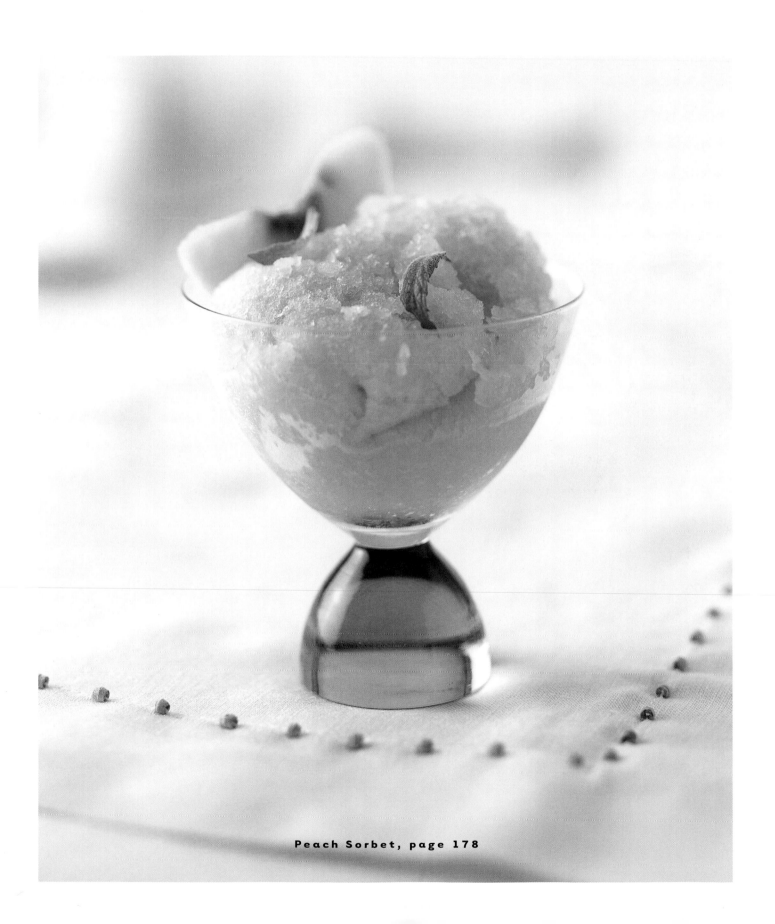

Peach Sorbet, page 178

Poached Summer Peaches with Cherries

In many areas, open-air markets and roadside stands abound with juicy, ripe peaches and sweet, tree-ripened cherries in late summer. Celebrate the bounty with this elegant dessert.

Exchanges: 1½ Fruit, ½ Fat

Nutrition Facts per serving: 142 cal., 4 g total fat (2 g sat. fat), 3 mg chol., 13 mg sodium, 17 g carbo., 2 g fiber, 1 g pro.
Daily Values: 4% vit. A, 10% vit. C, 1% calcium, 2% iron

1½ cups white Zinfandel, rosé wine, or cranberry-apple drink

1 2-inch piece stick cinnamon

3 medium peaches, halved and pitted

½ cup fresh dark or light sweet cherries (such as Bing or Rainier), pitted

2 ounces white baking bar

½ teaspoon shortening

Start to Finish: 30 minutes
Makes 6 servings

ONE In a 10-inch skillet bring wine and cinnamon just to boiling. Add peach halves and cherries; reduce heat. Simmer, covered, about 10 minutes or just until peaches are tender. Use a slotted spoon to transfer fruit to a shallow serving dish. **TWO** Cook the wine mixture, uncovered, over medium heat about 10 minutes or until reduced to about ½ cup. Discard cinnamon. Spoon the wine mixture over the peaches and cherries. **THREE** Meanwhile, in a small microwave-safe bowl microwave the baking bar and shortening on 100% power (high) for 1 to 1½ minutes or until melted, stirring once. Cool slightly. **FOUR** Spoon the melted baking bar into a self-sealing plastic bag. Snip a ¼-inch corner off the bottom of bag. Squeezing gently, drizzle the melted baking bar over the peaches and cherries.

Berries with Zabaglione

Keep this recipe handy for the fleeting fresh berry season. The rest of the year, spoon the rich, Marsala-flavored custard over a package of thawed, frozen unsweetened mixed fruit.

Exchanges: 1½ Fruit, 1 Fat

Nutrition Facts per serving: 136 cal., 5 g total fat (2 g sat. fat), 61 mg chol., 48 mg sodium, 19 g carbo., 2 g fiber, 4 g pro.
Daily Values: 11% vit. A, 27% vit. C, 12% calcium, 4% iron

---

2   tablespoons sugar

2   teaspoons cornstarch

¾   cup fat-free milk

1   beaten egg

¼   cup light dairy sour cream

2   tablespoons sweet or dry Marsala

2   cups berries (such as raspberries, blackberries, blueberries, and/or halved strawberries)

Ground cinnamon or nutmeg

Prep: 15 minutes
Chill: 2 hours
Makes 4 servings

ONE For custard, in a heavy medium saucepan combine sugar and cornstarch. Stir in milk. Cook and stir over medium heat until mixture is thickened and bubbly. Cook and stir for 2 minutes more. Remove from heat. **TWO** Gradually stir about half of the hot mixture into the beaten egg. Return all of the egg mixture to the saucepan. Cook until nearly bubbly, but do not boil. Immediately pour custard into a medium bowl; stir in sour cream and Marsala. Cover the surface with plastic wrap. Refrigerate for 2 to 24 hours. **THREE** To serve, divide the berries among 4 dessert dishes. Spoon the custard over the berries. Sprinkle with cinnamon. Serve immediately.

Mango and Raspberry Tart

Thanks to fat-free cream cheese, the filling in this low-fat dessert tastes deceptively rich. Another time, top the tart with sliced peaches or nectarines and blueberries.

Exchanges: ½ Fruit, 1 Starch, ½ Fat

Nutrition Facts per serving: 152 cal., 4 g total fat (3 g sat. fat), 14 mg chol., 90 mg sodium, 25 g carbo., 2 g fiber, 4 g pro.
Daily Values: 30% vit. A, 26% vit. C, 7% calcium, 3% iron

1	cup all-purpose flour
1	tablespoon sugar
¼	teaspoon salt
¼	cup butter
3	to 4 tablespoons cold water
1	8-ounce package fat-free cream cheese, softened
¼	cup sugar
1	teaspoon vanilla
1	26-ounce jar refrigerated mango slices, drained and chopped, or 2 cups chopped, peeled mangoes (2 medium)
1	cup fresh raspberries
½	cup low-calorie apricot spread

Prep: 40 minutes
Chill: 2 hours
Makes 12 servings

ONE In a medium bowl combine flour, the 1 tablespoon sugar, and the salt. Using a pastry blender, cut in butter until pieces are pea-size. Sprinkle 1 tablespoon of the water over part of the mixture; gently toss with a fork. Push moistened dough to side of bowl. Repeat using 1 tablespoon of the water at a time, until all of the dough is moistened. Form into a ball. **TWO** On a lightly floured surface, flatten dough. Roll from center to edges into a 12-inch circle. Ease into a 10-inch tart pan with a removable bottom, being careful not to stretch pastry. Press pastry up the side of pan. Trim pastry even with rim of pan. Prick the bottom well with a fork. Bake in a 450° oven for 12 to 15 minutes or until golden brown. Cool on a wire rack. **THREE** Meanwhile, in a medium mixing bowl combine the cream cheese, the ¼ cup sugar, and the vanilla. Beat with an electric mixer on medium speed until smooth. Spread over the cooled pastry. Arrange the mangoes in a 3-inch ring around the edge of the tart. Fill the center with raspberries. **FOUR** In a small saucepan heat the apricot spread until melted; cut up any large pieces. Spoon the melted spread over fruit. Refrigerate for 2 to 3 hours. Before serving, remove sides of pan.

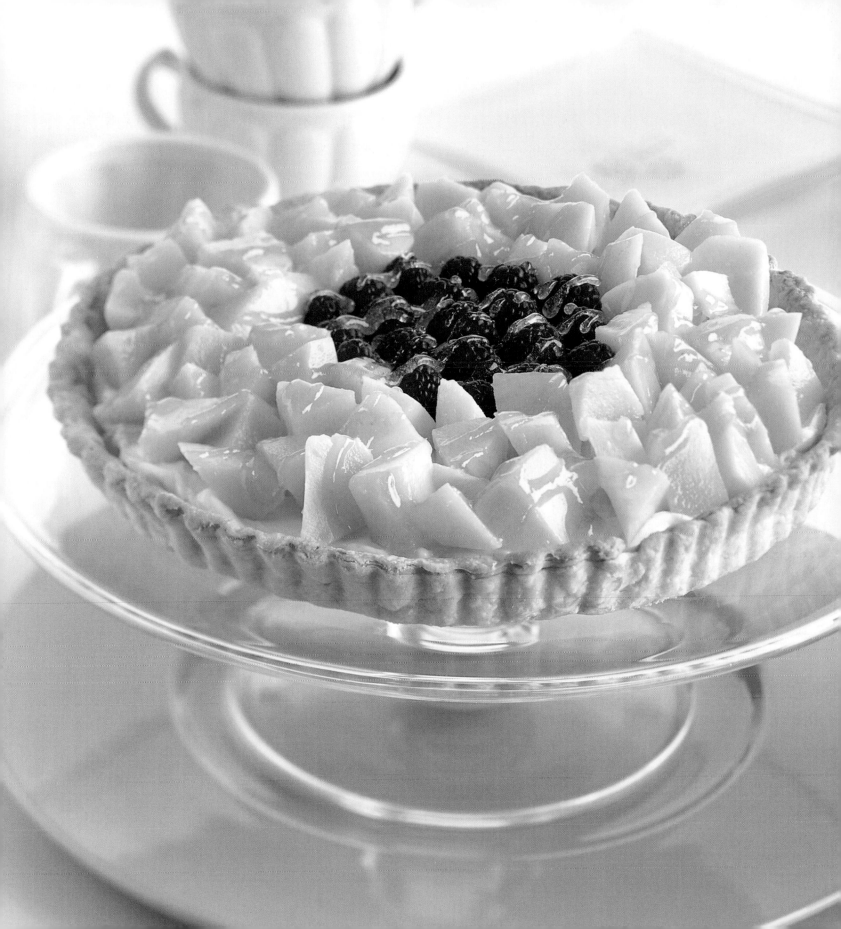

Cocoa-Nutmeg Snickerdoodles

You'll recognize this deliciously lightened version of an old-fashioned cookie by the familiar crinkled tops. The dusting of cocoa powder gives just a hint of chocolate flavor.

Exchanges: 1 Fat

Nutrition Facts per cookie: 51 cal., 1 g total fat (1 g sat. fat), 8 mg chol., 30 mg sodium, 9 g carbo., 0 g fiber, 1 g pro.
Daily Values: 1% vit. A, 1% calcium, 1% iron

⅓ cup butter

1 cup sugar

1 teaspoon baking powder

½ teaspoon ground nutmeg

¼ teaspoon baking soda

⅓ cup fat-free dairy sour cream

1 slightly beaten egg

1 teaspoon vanilla

2 cups all-purpose flour

Nonstick cooking spray

2 tablespoons sugar

1½ teaspoons unsweetened cocoa powder

Prep: 25 minutes
Chill: 1 hour
Bake: 10 minutes per batch
Makes about 48 cookies

ONE In a large bowl beat the butter with an electric mixer on medium to high speed for 30 seconds. Add the 1 cup sugar, the baking powder, nutmeg, and baking soda; beat until combined. Beat in the sour cream, egg, and vanilla until combined. Beat in as much of the flour as you can with the mixer. Stir in any remaining flour with a wooden spoon. Cover and refrigerate for 1 to 2 hours or until dough is easy to handle. **TWO** Lightly coat a cookie sheet with cooking spray; set aside. In a small bowl combine the 2 tablespoons sugar and the cocoa powder. Shape dough into 1-inch balls. Roll the balls in the cocoa mixture to coat. Place 2 inches apart on the prepared cookie sheet. **THREE** Bake in a 375° oven for 10 to 11 minutes or until edges are golden brown. Transfer cookies to a wire rack; cool completely.

Gossamer Spice Cookies

A bevy of traditional dessert spices with just a bit of rambunctious red pepper gives these extra-thin, extra-crisp cookies an old-world flavor. Serve them with a fruit sorbet for a pleasing contrast of flavor and texture.

Exchanges: ½ Fat

Nutrition Facts per cookie: 25 cal., 1 g total fat (0 g sat. fat), 1 mg chol., 9 mg sodium, 4 g carbo., 0 g fiber, 0 g pro.
Daily Values: 1% iron

⅓	cup butter
¼	cup packed dark brown sugar
½	teaspoon ground ginger
½	teaspoon apple pie spice
¼	teaspoon ground cloves
¼	teaspoon ground cardamom
⅛	teaspoon ground red pepper
⅓	cup molasses
1⅓	cups all-purpose flour

Prep: 35 minutes
Chill: 1 hour
Bake: 5 minutes per batch
Makes about 66 cookies

ONE In a large bowl beat the butter with an electric mixer on medium to high speed for 30 seconds. Add the brown sugar, ginger, apple pie spice, cloves, cardamom, and red pepper; beat until combined. Beat in the molasses until combined. Beat in as much of the flour as you can with the mixer. Stir in any remaining flour with a wooden spoon. Divide dough in half. Cover and refrigerate about 1 hour or until dough is easy to handle. **TWO** On a lightly floured surface, roll each portion of dough to ¹⁄₁₆-inch thickness. Cut with a 2-inch scalloped round cookie or biscuit cutter. Place on an ungreased cookie sheet. **THREE** Bake in a 375° oven for 5 to 6 minutes or until edges are browned. Transfer cookies to a wire rack; cool completely.

Sugar Scoop

Be aware that other sweeteners—such as honey, maple syrup, or corn syrup—might not be better for you than ordinary sugar. Nutritionally speaking, they are all much the same. Sugar does not garner high nutrition points. In a healthful diet, sweets should be considered a treat and eaten in moderation. Follow your eating plan and work dessert in when you can, without making a habit of substituting cookie calories for fruits, veggies, and whole grains.

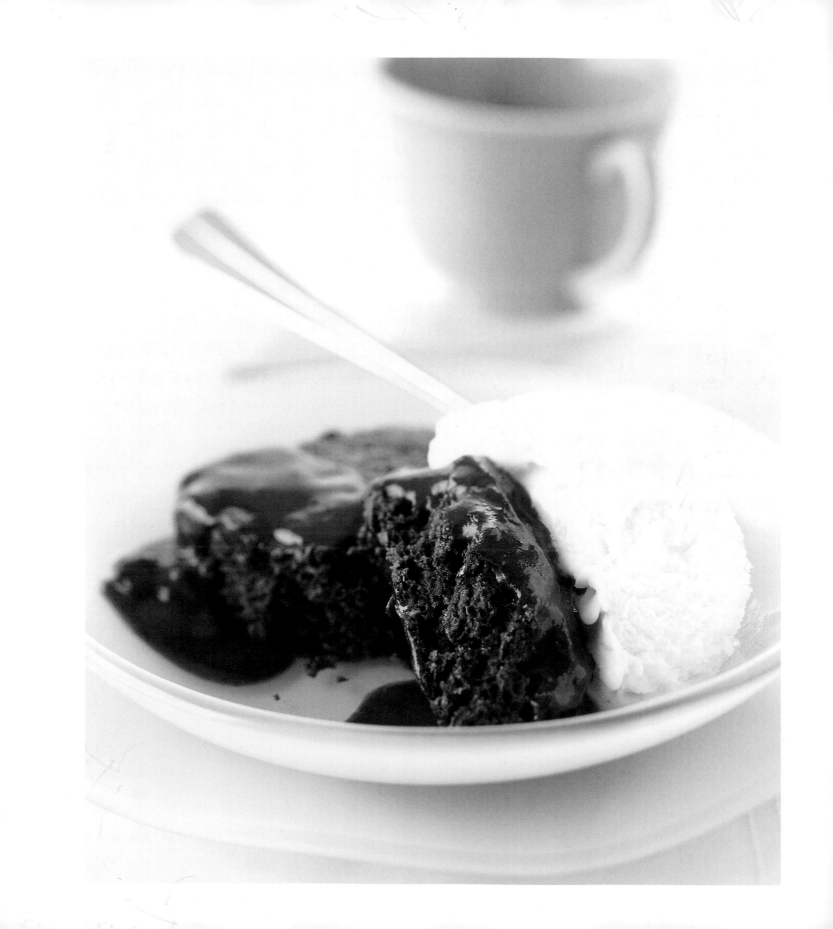

Mocha Pudding Cake

Butter might make batter better, but in this moist, gooey cake, applesauce replaces the butter and keeps the dessert slim and trim. Serve it warm and topped with fresh nectarine slices or berries.

Exchanges: 2 Starch, 2 Fat

Nutrition Facts per serving: 242 cal., 1 g total fat (0 g sat. fat), 0 mg chol., 264 mg sodium, 56 g carbo., 1 g fiber, 3 g pro.
Daily Values: 1% vit. A, 1% vit. C, 16% calcium, 10% iron

Nonstick cooking spray

1 cup all-purpose flour

¾ cup granulated sugar

¼ cup unsweetened cocoa powder

2 teaspoons baking powder

½ teaspoon salt

½ cup fat-free milk

½ cup applesauce

1 teaspoon vanilla

1¾ cups hot water

¾ cup packed brown sugar

¼ cup unsweetened cocoa powder

1 teaspoon instant coffee crystals

Nonfat frozen yogurt (optional)

Prep: 20 minutes
Bake: 45 minutes
Makes 8 to 10 servings

ONE Lightly coat an 8×8×2-inch baking pan with cooking spray; set aside. In a large bowl combine the flour, granulated sugar, ¼ cup cocoa powder, the baking powder, and salt. Stir in milk, applesauce, and vanilla until well combined. Spread batter in the prepared baking pan. **TWO** In a medium bowl combine the hot water, brown sugar, ¼ cup cocoa powder, and the coffee crystals. Carefully pour the coffee mixture over the cake batter. **THREE** Bake in a 350° oven about 45 minutes or until a wooden toothpick inserted near the center comes out clean. Cool slightly on a wire rack. Spoon the warm cake and pudding into dessert dishes. If desired, serve with frozen yogurt.

Oatmeal-Applesauce Cake

The combination of applesauce, raisins, and spices gives your kitchen a heavenly scent while this cake bakes. Serve the sugar-sprinkled squares with mugs of steaming coffee.

Exchanges: 1 Starch, 1 Fat

Nutrition Facts per serving: 151 cal., 4 g total fat (2 g sat. fat), 8 mg chol., 140 mg sodium, 29 g carbo., 1 g fiber, 2 g pro.

Nonstick cooking spray

2	cups all-purpose flour
²/₃	cup quick-cooking rolled oats
2	teaspoons baking powder
½	teaspoon baking soda
½	teaspoon ground cinnamon
¼	teaspoon salt
⅛	teaspoon ground nutmeg
⅓	cup butter
1	cup packed brown sugar
1¾	cups applesauce
¼	cup refrigerated or frozen egg product, thawed
1	teaspoon vanilla
¾	cup raisins or mixed dried fruit bits
1	tablespoon sifted powdered sugar

Prep: 15 minutes
Bake: 25 minutes
Cool: 2 hours
Makes 20 servings

ONE Lightly coat a 13×9×2-inch baking pan with cooking spray; set aside. In a medium bowl stir together the flour, oats, baking powder, baking soda, cinnamon, salt, and nutmeg. Set aside. **TWO** In a large bowl beat the butter with an electric mixer on medium to high speed for 30 seconds. Add the brown sugar; beat until fluffy. Add the applesauce, egg product, and vanilla; beat until well combined. Add the flour mixture; beat until combined. Stir in raisins. Spread batter in the prepared baking pan. **THREE** Bake in a 350° oven for 25 to 30 minutes or until a wooden toothpick inserted near the center comes out clean. Cool completely in pan on a wire rack. Sprinkle with powdered sugar.

Warm Chocolate Bread Pudding

This splendid orange-scented combination of chocolate and custard can easily be doubled to serve four. For a special touch, place the soufflé dishes on dessert plates lined with paper doilies.

Exchanges: 1 Starch, 1 Fat

Nutrition Facts per serving: 163 cal., 4 g total fat (0 g sat. fat), 0 mg chol., 125 mg sodium, 29 g carbo., 0 g fiber, 5 g pro.
Daily Values: 13% vit. A, 1% vit. C, 6% calcium, 7% iron

Nonstick cooking spray

1   cup firm-textured white bread cubes (about 1¼ slices of Italian or sourdough bread)

⅓   cup fat-free milk

2   tablespoons sugar

2   tablespoons miniature semisweet chocolate pieces

3   tablespoons refrigerated or frozen egg product, thawed, or 1 egg

½   teaspoon finely shredded orange or tangerine peel

¼   teaspoon vanilla

Sifted powdered sugar or fat-free pressurized whipped dessert topping (optional)

Prep: 25 minutes
Bake: 15 minutes
Makes 2 servings

ONE Coat two 6-ounce individual soufflé dishes or custard cups with nonstick cooking spray. Divide the bread cubes between the prepared dishes. **TWO** In a small saucepan combine the milk, sugar, and chocolate pieces. Cook and stir over low heat until chocolate is melted. Remove from heat. If necessary, use a wire whisk to beat until smooth. **THREE** In a small bowl combine the egg product, orange peel, and vanilla. Gradually stir in the chocolate mixture. Pour over the bread cubes in dishes. Press lightly with the back of a spoon to thoroughly moisten bread. If desired, cover and refrigerate for up to 2 hours before baking. **FOUR** Bake, uncovered, in a 350° oven for 15 to 20 minutes or until the tops appear firm and a knife inserted near centers comes out clean. Cool slightly on a wire rack. If desired, sprinkle the warm puddings with powdered sugar.

Chocolate—A Source of Antioxidants?

That's right. Chocolate is a plant-based food—not that it should replace fruits and vegetables in your diet—but it can be an enjoyable, healthful addition. In fact, chocolate contains flavonoids that act as powerful antioxidants. These antioxidants squelch free radicals and have a role in protecting your heart by preventing the accumulation of fat in the arteries. Even more noteworthy, while chocolate is known for its high saturated fat content, the fat in chocolate appears to have a neutral, or even slightly positive effect on lowering cholesterol.

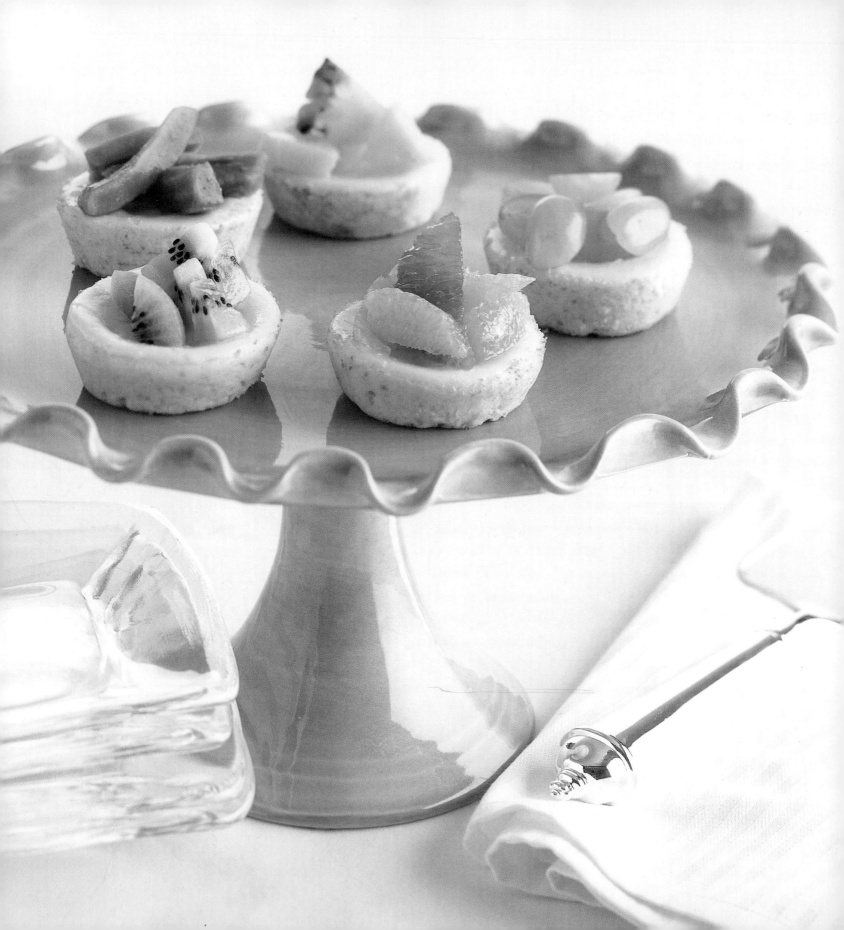

Mini Cheesecakes

Just a couple of bites each, these tiny cheesecakes burst with flavor and satisfy any sweet tooth. To create a colorful party platter, top the miniature desserts with an assortment of fresh fruits.

Exchanges: 1 Starch, 1 Fat

Nutrition Facts per serving: 124 cal., 4 g total fat (1 g sat. fat), 5 mg chol., 25 mg sodium, 16 g carbo., 0 g fiber, 6 g pro.
Daily Values: 13% vit. A, 10% vit. C, 10% calcium, 1% iron

Nonstick cooking spray

⅓ cup crushed vanilla wafers (about 8 wafers)

1½ 8-ounce tubs fat-free cream cheese, softened (12 ounces total)

½ cup sugar

1 tablespoon all-purpose flour

1 teaspoon vanilla

¼ cup refrigerated or frozen egg product, thawed

¾ cup fresh fruit (such as halved grapes, cut-up pineapple, cut-up peeled kiwifruit or papaya, red raspberries, blueberries, sliced strawberries, sliced plums, and/or orange and grapefruit sections)

Prep: 20 minutes
Bake: 18 minutes
Chill: 4 hours
Makes 10 cheesecakes

ONE Coat ten 2½-inch muffin cups with cooking spray. Sprinkle the bottom and side of each cup with a rounded teaspoon of the crushed vanilla wafers. Set aside. **TWO** In a medium bowl beat the cream cheese with an electric mixer on medium speed until smooth. Add sugar, flour, and vanilla. Beat on medium speed until smooth. Add egg product; beat on low speed just until combined. Divide evenly among the prepared muffin cups. **THREE** Bake in a 325° oven for 18 to 20 minutes or until set. Cool in muffin cups on a wire rack for 5 minutes. Cover and refrigerate for 4 to 24 hours. **FOUR** Remove the cheesecakes from muffin cups. Just before serving, top the cheesecakes with fresh fruit.

Peach Sorbet

This cool, refreshing treat makes the hottest days of summer more tolerable. Top scoops of sorbet with fresh peach slices and mint leaves for a simply stunning dessert (see photo, page 165).

Exchanges: 1 Fruit, 1 Starch

Nutrition Facts per serving: 141 cal., 0 g total fat (0 g sat. fat), 0 mg chol., 3 mg sodium, 32 g carbo., 1 g fiber, 0 g pro.
Daily Values: 2% vit. A, 11% vit. C, 1% iron

1¼ pounds peaches, peeled and cut up (2½ cups) or one 16-ounce package frozen unsweetened peach slices, slightly thawed

3 tablespoons lemon juice

1 cup sugar

1 cup boiling water

1 cup dry white wine

1½ teaspoons finely shredded orange peel

Peach slices (optional)

Small mint leaves (optional)

Prep: 20 minutes
Freeze: 9 hours
Stand: 20 minutes
Makes 8 servings

ONE In a blender container or food processor bowl combine the peaches and lemon juice. Cover and blend or process until smooth. **TWO** In a large bowl combine the sugar and boiling water; stir until sugar is dissolved. Stir in the peach mixture, wine, and orange peel. Pour into a 9×9×2-inch pan. **THREE** Cover and freeze for 3 to 4 hours or until firm. Break into chunks; transfer to a chilled large bowl. Beat with an electric mixer on medium to high speed until smooth. Return to pan. Cover and freeze at least 6 hours or until firm. Before serving, let stand at room temperature for 20 minutes. If desired, garnish with peach slices and mint leaves.

Espresso Granita

The slightly bitter, slightly rich flavor of coffee explodes from this cool, icy dessert. If needed, substitute 3 cups of cold water mixed with 3 tablespoons instant espresso powder for the strong brewed espresso in the recipe.

Exchanges: 1 Starch

Nutrition Facts per serving: 50 cal., 0 g total fat (0 g sat. fat), 0 mg chol., 3 mg sodium, 13 g carbo., 0 g fiber, 0 g pro.

1	cup water
½	cup sugar
3	cups strong brewed espresso, cooled
1	teaspoon anisette liqueur (optional)

Prep: 15 minutes
Stand: 5 minutes
Cool: 30 minutes
Freeze: 10½ hours
Makes 8 servings

ONE In a medium saucepan combine the water and sugar. Cook and stir over medium heat until sugar is dissolved. Remove from heat; cool about 30 minutes. Stir in the espresso and, if desired, anisette liqueur. Pour into a 13×9×2-inch pan. **TWO** Cover and freeze about 1½ hours or until mixture is slushy at the edges. Stir, scraping the frozen mixture off the bottom and sides of the pan. Cover and freeze for 3 to 3½ hours or until all of the mixture is slushy, stirring every 30 minutes. Cover and freeze for at least 6 hours or until firm. **THREE** Before serving, let stand at room temperature for 15 to 10 minutes. Scrape the surface of the granita and spoon into chilled dessert dishes.

exercise.101

Perhaps you've seen those magazine ads that boast, "Lose weight without breaking a sweat!" or you've heard the woman over the radio testify, "I lost weight and didn't move a muscle!" You might even know someone who was able to slim down without hitting the gym. Yet numerous books, magazines, and weight loss experts insist that permanent weight loss is nearly impossible without regular physical activity.

Why is exercise important to successful weight control? Simply stated, exercise burns calories, so it tips the scales in your favor for weight loss. For example, if you eat the same amount of calories as you burn through exercise or daily activities, you will maintain your weight. If you burn more calories than you eat, you will lose weight.

Maintaining or building muscle mass is an added benefit of exercise. Muscle is more metabolically active than fat tissue. Muscles burn energy and require calories to maintain their size, even when you aren't using them. If you lose muscle, you lose tissue that helps you burn calories. Loss of muscle has a direct negative effect on your ability to lose weight and keep it off. Unfortunately, dieting results in the loss of muscle as well as fat. How do you prevent excessive loss of muscle while dieting? **Exercise!**

Exercise also has the potential to improve your mental well-being. Consistent exercisers have less anxiety and depression. By increasing your sense of personal control, buffering your body's reaction to stress, and enhancing self-esteem, exercise proves invaluable to the mind and body undergoing a weight loss program. The single greatest predictor of successful weight loss maintenance is exercise, as 80 percent of maintainers are regular, consistent exercisers.

Regular physical activity is fun and healthful. For most people, increasing their activity level is safe. However, some people should check with a doctor before becoming more physically active.

If you're planning to become more physically active than you are now, answer the following seven questions. The PAR-Q & You questionnaire (as adapted from Thomas, Reading, and Shephard) can determine readiness for exercise. If you're between the ages of 15 and 69, the PAR-Q will tell you if you should check with your doctor before you start. If you're more than 69 years of age, and you're not used to being active, check with your doctor first.

Common sense is your best guide when you answer these questions. Read the questions carefully and answer each honestly.

Check YES or NO:

<u>Y</u>/<u>N</u> Has your doctor ever said that you have a heart condition and that you should only do physical activity recommended by a doctor?

<u>Y</u>/<u>N</u> Do you feel pain in your chest when you do physical activity?

<u>Y</u>/<u>N</u> In the past month, have you had chest pain when you were not doing physical activity?

<u>Y</u>/<u>N</u> Do you lose your balance because of dizziness or do you ever lose consciousness?

<u>Y</u>/<u>N</u> Do you have a bone or joint problem that could be made worse by a change in your physical activity?

<u>Y</u>/N Is your doctor currently prescribing drugs (for example, water pills) for a blood pressure or heart condition?

<u>Y</u>/<u>N</u> Do you know of any other reason why you should not do physical activity?

If you answered YES to one or more questions, talk with your doctor before you become more physically active or before you have a fitness appraisal. Tell your doctor about the PAR-Q and which questions you answered YES. You might be able to do any activity you want as long as you start slowly and progress gradually, or you may need to restrict your activities. Talk to your doctor about the kinds of activities you wish to do, and follow his or her advice. Find out which community programs are safe and helpful for you.

If you answered NO honestly to all PAR-Q questions, you can be reasonably sure that you can safely become more physically active. Begin slowly and build gradually. This is the safest and easiest way to go. Take part in a fitness appraisal. This is an excellent way to determine your basic fitness level so you can plan the best way to live actively.

Delay becoming more active if you are not feeling well because of a temporary illness such as a cold or a fever—wait until you feel better. Also, if you are or may become pregnant, talk to your doctor before you become more active.

Finally, if your health changes so that you answer YES to any of the above questions, tell your fitness or health professional. Ask whether you should change your physical activity plan.

Choosing the Best Exercise Program

Does your treadmill double as a clothes hanger? Exhausted after a long day at work, do you zoom right past the gym on the ride home? Are you finding it hard to cross the threshold of intention to actually exercise? Try to approach exercise from a different angle. Exercise can be fun—it doesn't have to be painful to be beneficial. If you have the green light from your doctor to work up a little sweat, consider the following questions when considering what types of exercise to try:

• **How much extra time are you willing and able to devote to exercise?**

• **What are your resources: home exercise equipment, fitness club memberships, community-based classes, accessibility and safety of neighborhood sidewalks and parks?**

• **Do you enjoy independent exercise or the company of others?**

• **What activities do you enjoy or have you enjoyed in the past?**

Whether you seek professional advice from a certified exercise physiologist or a certified personal trainer, or personally initiate a plan, it is important to understand the differences between the two forms of exercise most relevant to weight loss: cardiovascular exercise (e.g., aerobic exercise) and resistance training (e.g., weight lifting). Cardiovascular exercise is any activity requiring continuous movement that places a high demand on the body's heart, lungs, and muscles. Walking, bicycling, aerobic dance, deep-water jogging, kickboxing, and cycling are all forms of cardiovascular exercise. Besides being a great weight loss tool, cardiovascular exercise increases serum HDL (good) cholesterol levels, helps your body use insulin efficiently, and rids the body of damaging free radicals. As a consequence, people who participate in regular cardiovascular exercise have a decreased risk of heart disease, diabetes, and even certain forms of cancer!

Resistance training includes exercises that increase muscle size and strength. The good news for women, aside from some ability to build muscle, is that resistance training increases bone density and reduces the risk of osteoporosis.

For optimal weight loss, it's best to include both types of exercise. Research from the National Weight Loss Registry describes the successful weight loss maintainer as someone who performs four to five hours of cardiovascular exercise weekly.

While it is obviously important to select activities that you enjoy, other considerations that affect the appropriate type of exercise include existing muscle or joint pain or injuries that prevent high-impact activity such as running, or mobility restrictions from pain or excess body weight. Many overweight exercisers find that while weight-bearing activity such as walking is difficult, the same movement in water is virtually pain-free. From Arthritis Foundation-sponsored aquatic aerobic classes to deep-water jogging, your local department of recreation, community college, or fitness club may offer aquatic programs worth checking out.

Start it up!

Before you actually get going, it is important to understand some exercise lingo. **Frequency** refers to the number of days per week dedicated to exercise. **Duration** is the amount of time spent per session. **Intensity** is how hard you work.

Your heart rate, measured by your pulse, is the best way to follow your exercise intensity. Find your pulse by placing your index and middle fingers at either the carotid (neck) or the radial (wrist) artery. Count the number of beats in 10 seconds. Multiply that number by six. For example, if you counted 12 beats in 10 seconds, your heart rate is 72 beats per minute.

Once you've learned how to monitor your heart rate, you can calculate your target heart rate zone. This is the range of intensity that promotes safe cardiovascular improvement. As with determining your calorie needs, it's necessary to do a little math to find your target heart rate zone. For safety, this target zone will be less than the maximum heart rate you are capable of achieving (estimated by subtracting your age from 220). To determine your zone, choose the category that best describes your current activity level (beginner or intermediate exerciser). Follow the examples for the appropriate category:

BEGINNER LOW END

(if you haven't participated in regular activity within the last 6 months)

(220 minus your age) multiplied by 60 percent

e.g.: (220 - 50 years) x 0.60 = 102 beats/minute

INTERMEDIATE LOW END

(if you currently exercise)

(220 minus your age) multiplied by 70 percent

e.g.: (220 - 50 years) x 0.70 = 119 beats/minute

BOTH LEVELS HIGH END

(220 minus your age) multiplied by 85 percent

e.g.: (220 - 50 years) x 0.85 = 144 beats/minute

For example, a 50-year-old beginner's target heart zone is 102 to 144 beats per minute. A 50-year-old intermediate's target heart rate zone is 119 to 144 beats per minute. **Be honest and conservative when calculating your zone!** If you are a beginner, your current endurance can't sustain exercise intensity much beyond 60 percent, so start easily. With every exercise session your body will adapt and grow stronger. Over time you will notice that your heart doesn't have to work as hard even though your intensity is the same. Perhaps brisk walking at a 3.0 mph pace initially elicited a heart rate of 110 beats per minute. Two weeks later, the same pace might produce a heart rate of 100 beats per minute. Your heart has positively adapted by producing the same volume of exercise for less effort! This is your green light to increase your pace within your target heart rate zone.

Exercise physiologists use the term **progression** when prescribing exercise programs. To begin an exercise program, over a period of time you must slowly increase the frequency, duration, and intensity. The following table maps out a 15-week plan of safe and effective exercise progression:

Week	Frequency	Intensity	Duration
	(Sessions/Week)	(% Max Heart Rate)	(minutes/session)
1	3	60	15-20
2-4	3-4	60-70	18-23
5-8	3-4	70-80	21-26
9-11	3-4	70-80	24-29
12-14	3-4	70-85	27-32
15+	4-5	70-85	30-45

Four Steps to Exercise

In a group exercise class, the instructor takes you through a series of four phases necessary for injury prevention. If you are exercising independently, you must work through these phases on your own.

ONE. Warm-up The first 5 to 10 minutes of any activity should include similar movements at an intensity slightly below your target heart range. For example, if treadmill walking at a 4.0 mph pace produces a heart rate equal to 70 percent of your training target zone, start walking at a 3.0 mph pace, gradually building speed. The purpose of the warm-up is to gradually increase your body's core temperature and blood flow to working muscles.

TWO. Workout Seventy percent of your total exercise duration should be spent here, in your target heart rate zone. When you increase the duration of exercise (as previously outlined), the workout portion is the part that lengthens.

THREE. Cool down Suddenly stopping exercise while within your target heart rate zone is the equivalent of driving your car at 55 mph and pulling up on the emergency brake. Like the warm-up, the last 5 to 10 minutes of your session should include slower movements that return blood from the working muscles to the heart, preventing any pooling of blood in your lower extremities. You want to feel good after your workout, not faint, so be sure to gradually cool down.

FOUR. Stretch Because stretching a previously inactive muscle is like pulling on a cold rubber band (think "snap"), stretching should ALWAYS FOLLOW and NEVER PRECEDE an exercise session. Taking an extra 5 to 10 minutes after your workout to stretch increases muscle flexibility and prevents injury and soreness.

Maintenance

How to Adapt Your Plan After Weight Loss

Congratulations! Now that you have achieved your goal weight, don't let that hard work go down the drain. Sometimes sustaining your weight loss is the trickiest part. People often make the mistake of considering their new, more healthful habits as temporary, to be discontinued once they reach their goal weight. The most important thing to remember in order to maintain your weight loss is to continue doing whatever helped you lose weight, indefinitely! If Nike's motto for life is "Just Do It!" our motto at the Johns Hopkins Weight

Management Center is "Just Keep Doing It!"

If you stop paying attention to your eating and exercise behavior, your weight is likely to come back. Be aware of the changes in your lifestyle that helped you achieve a healthier weight. Work to maintain these changes even after weight loss! If giving up or reducing fast food helped you lose weight, then this same strategy should help you keep the weight off. If you found keeping a food journal to be useful, continue using it even after you've achieved your weight loss goal. Remember the tools that helped you reach your goal.

Weighing yourself at least weekly is also important so you can make adjustments in your eating or activity level if you regain even a few pounds. Establish a maximum weight gain that is acceptable to you and actions to take if you pass this limit. It is always better to deal with small weight gains before the pounds become seemingly insurmountable. If you don't weigh yourself regularly, select an article of clothing that will help you monitor changes in your weight.

If you maintain your current exercise program, you will be able to eat a fair amount and still keep off your weight. Adjust the caloric level of your eating plan to maintain your weight. Retrace the three steps for determining calorie needs using your new activity level and weight. Don't subtract any calories for weight loss; instead, use this new calorie level to maintain your weight.

If you stop or decrease your exercise regimen, the story changes. Gradual weight gain after weight loss is often more a consequence of less physical activity than of significant increases in food intake. Regular activity, even something as simple as walking, is the best predictor of long-term weight maintenance. Keep moving!

Champions For Your Cause

Choosing Appropriate Support Systems

Finally, ongoing support from a professional support group or your physician may be extremely beneficial in helping you achieve long-term maintenance of your weight loss. Other means of support are available through books such as this one, local support networks, weight management programs (e.g., TOPS and Weight Watchers), and friends or relatives who will follow a weight control program with you. Aim for supporting one another's efforts instead of competing. Another means of support may include internet discussion groups. Visit the Better Homes and Gardens Weight Loss Success discussion group at www.bhg.com for encouragement and understanding.

Most important, have clear, long-range goals in each of the areas emphasized in this book: diet, behavior, and exercise. Monitor your progress and your maintenance closely. You've invested time and effort in your new lifestyle. Have confidence in your ability to achieve your goals, and the results will follow.

Enjoy both the process (made easier with the delicious recipes in this book) and the results!

Progress Journal

Name _____ **Date** _____ **Weight** _____

<u>Water</u> **Each number represents one 8-ounce glass of water. Cross them off as you drink them throughout the day.**

    1   2   3   4   5   6   7   8   9

<u>Eating Log</u> **(Use the Food Lists on pages 12-13, or nutritional information listed with each recipe to estimate calories.)**

Time	Food or Beverage	Amount	Calories	Place, Motivation, Emotion

<u>**Daily Calorie Intake =**</u> _____

Physical Activity

Time	Activity	Duration

1,200 Calorie Sample Menu

Monday

Breakfast
Fruited
Granola
(page 25)

banana,
1 small

vanilla low-fat
yogurt, 1 cup

hot tea

Lunch
Muffuletta
(page 97)

green grapes,
½ cup

baby carrots,
1 cup

fat-free milk,
1 cup

Dinner
Pork
Medallions
with Pear
Sauce
(page 77)

steamed
asparagus,
8 spears

Wheat and Oat
Bread
(page 156)

margarine,
1 tablespoon

Espresso
Granita
(page 179)

fat-free milk,
1 cup

Snack
Energy Bar
(page 40)

Tuesday

Breakfast
The Casual
Omelet
(page 24)

whole wheat
toast, 1 slice

apricot
preserves,
1 tablespoon

vanilla soy
milk, 1 cup

orange juice,
¾ cup

Lunch
Gazpacho
Sandwich to
Go (page 140)

honeydew
melon, 1 cup

pretzel twists,
¼ cup

sparkling
bottled water

Dinner
Summer
Chicken and
Mushroom
Pasta (page 88)

baby greens,
1 cup

fat-free
dressing,
1 tablespoon

fat-free milk,
1 cup

Peach Sorbet
(page 178)

Snack
fat-free lemon
yogurt, 1 cup
berries, ½ cup
vanilla wafers, 2

Wednesday

Breakfast
toasted
cinnamon-
raisin bagel,
1 small

light cream
cheese
(Neufchâtel),
2 tablespoons

cantaloupe,
1 cup

fat-free milk,
1 cup

hot tea

Lunch
Chopped
Salmon Salad
(page 59)

crisp
breadsticks, 2

fresh plums,
2 small

club soda

Dinner
Beef Satay with
Spicy Peanut
Sauce
(page 68)

long grain rice,
½ cup

grilled
zucchini and
summer
squash, sliced,
1 cup

fat-free milk,
1 cup

Snack
reduced-fat
cheddar
cheese, 1 oz.

whole wheat
crackers, 5

Thursday

Breakfast
Breakfast Rice
Cereal
(page 28)

whole grain
English
muffin,
2 halves

honey,
1 tablespoon

fat-free milk,
1 cup.

Lunch
Chicken-
Zucchini Salad
(page 56)

plum
tomatoes,
sliced, 2

toasted
sourdough
bread,
1 slice

sparkling
water

Dinner
Baked Salmon
and Vegetables
(page 114)

broccoli, ½ cup

baked potato,
1 small

margarine,
2 teaspoons

iced tea

Snack
Super Soy
Smoothie
(page 33)

Friday

Breakfast
Tropical Coffee
Cake (page 30)

papaya,
½ small

coffee

Lunch
ham on rye:
2 oz. ham
1 oz. reduced-
fat Swiss
cheese
2 slices rye
bread
lettuce,
tomato,
mustard

nectarine,
1 small

fat-free milk,
1 cup

Dinner
Three-
Cheese-
Stuffed Shells
(page 127)

torn romaine,
1½ cups with
fat-free
dressing

Easy Herb
Focaccia
(page 157)

fat-free milk,
1 cup

Snack
Vegetable
Spring Rolls 2
(page 38)

Saturday

Breakfast
Breakfast
Bread Pudding
(page 27)

orange juice,
¾ cup

hot tea

Lunch
Shrimp
Gazpacho
(page 123)

sparkling
water

Cocoa Nutmeg
Snickerdoodle,
1 cookie
(page 170)

Dinner
Roast Tarragon
Chicken
(page 94)

mashed
potatoes,
½ cup

steamed green
beans, ¾ cup

whole grain
bread, 1 slice

margarine,
2 teaspoons

fat-free milk,
1 cup

Snack
Strawberries
with Lime
Dipping Sauce
(page 45)

Sunday

Brunch
Cheddar-
Polenta Puff
(page 21)

Spinach-
Apricot Salad
(page 152)

mini bran
muffins, 2

Berries with
Zabaglione
(page 167)

coffee

Dinner
Horseradish
Flank Steak
(page 67)

Orange-
Ginger Carrots
(page 149)

Hearty Bulgur
Pilaf
(page 161)

crusty French
roll, 1

fat-free milk,
1 cup

Snack
iced chocolate
soy milk,
1½ cups

Index

Photographs indicated in bold.

Metric Cooking Hints

By making a few conversions, cooks in Australia, Canada, and the United Kingdom can use the recipes in this book with confidence. The charts on this page provide a guide for converting measurements from the U.S. customary system, which is used throughout this book, to the imperial and metric systems. There also is a conversion table for oven temperatures to accommodate the differences in oven calibrations.

Product Differences: Most of the ingredients called for in the recipes in this book are available in English-speaking countries. However, some are known by different names. Here are some common U.S. American ingredients and their possible counterparts:

- Sugar is granulated or castor sugar.

- Powdered sugar is icing sugar.

- All-purpose flour is plain household flour or white flour. When self-rising flour is used in place of all-purpose flour in a recipe that calls for leavening, omit the leavening agent (baking soda or baking powder) and salt.

- Light-colored corn syrup is golden syrup.

- Cornstarch is cornflour.

- Baking soda is bicarbonate of soda.

- Vanilla is vanilla essence.

- Green, red, or yellow sweet peppers are capsicums.

- Golden raisins are sultanas.

Volume and Weight: U.S. Americans traditionally use cup measures for liquid and solid ingredients. The chart, below, shows the approximate imperial and metric equivalents. If you are accustomed to weighing solid ingredients, the following approximate equivalents will help.

- 1 cup butter, castor sugar, or rice = 8 ounces = about 230 grams

- 1 cup flour = 4 ounces = about 115 grams

- 1 cup icing sugar = 5 ounces = about 140 grams

Spoon measures are used for smaller amounts of ingredients. Although the size of the tablespoon varies slightly in different countries, for practical purposes and for recipes in this book, a straight substitution is all that's necessary.

Measurements made using cups or spoons always should be level unless stated otherwise.

Equivalents: U.S. = Australia/U.K.

$\frac{1}{8}$ teaspoon = 1 ml
$\frac{1}{4}$ teaspoon = 1.25 ml
$\frac{1}{2}$ teaspoon = 2.5 ml
1 teaspoon = 5 ml
1 tablespoon = 15 ml
1 fluid ounce = 30 ml
$\frac{1}{4}$ cup = 60 ml
$\frac{1}{3}$ cup = 80 ml
$\frac{1}{2}$ cup = 120 ml
$\frac{2}{3}$ cup = 160 ml
$\frac{3}{4}$ cup = 180 ml
1 cup = 240 ml
2 cups = 475 ml
1 quart = 1 liter
$\frac{1}{2}$ inch = 1.25 cm
1 inch = 2.5 cm

Baking Pan Sizes

U.S.	Metric
8×1½-inch round baking pan	20×4-cm cake tin
9×1½-inch round baking pan	23×4-cm cake tin
11×7×1½-inch baking pan	28×18×4-cm baking tin
13×9×2-inch baking pan	32×23×5-cm baking tin
2-quart rectangular baking dish	28×18×4-cm baking tin
15×10×1-inch baking pan	38×25.5×2.5-cm baking tin (Swiss roll tin)
9-inch pie plate	22×4- or 23×4-cm pie plate
7- or 8-inch springform pan	18- or 20-cm springform or loose-bottom cake tin
9×5×3-inch loaf pan	23×13×8-cm or 2-pound narrow loaf tin or pâté tin
1½-quart casserole	1.5-liter casserole
2-quart casserole	2-liter casserole

Oven Temperature Equivalents

Fahrenheit Setting	Celsius Setting*	Gas Setting
300°F	150°C	Gas mark 2 (very low)
325°F	170°C	Gas mark 3 (low)
350°F	180°C	Gas mark 4 (moderate)
375°F	190°C	Gas mark 5 (moderately hot)
400°F	200°C	Gas mark 6 (hot)
425°F	220°C	Gas mark 7 (hot)
450°F	230°C	Gas mark 8 (very hot)
475°F	240°C	Gas mark 9 (very hot)
Broil		Grill

*Electric and gas ovens may be calibrated using Celsius. However, for an electric oven, increase the Celsius setting 10 to 20 degrees when cooking above 160°C. For convection or forced-air ovens (gas or electric), lower the temperature setting 10°C when cooking at all heat levels.